WHY
WON'T YOU
SLEEP?!

Also by Kim West, MSW

The Sleep Lady's Gentle Newborn Sleep Guide:
Trusted Solutions for Getting You and Your Baby FAST
to Sleep Without Leaving Them to Cry It Out

The Sleep Lady's Good Night, Sleep Tight:
Gentle Proven Solutions to Help Your Child Sleep
Without Leaving Them to Cry It Out

The Good Night, Sleep Tight Workbook: Gentle Proven Solutions
to Help Your Child Sleep Well and Wake Up Happy

The Good Night, Sleep Tight Workbook for Children with
Special Needs: Gentle Proven Solutions to Help Your Child
with Special Needs Sleep Well and Wake Up Happy
(with Katie Holloran)

The Newborn Twins Sleep Guide:
The Nap and Nighttime Sanity Saver for Your Duo's First Five Months
(with Natalie Diaz)

WHY
WON'T YOU
SLEEP?!

A Game-Changing Approach
for Exhausted Parents of Nonstop,
Super Alert, Big Feeling Kids

Macall Gordon, MA, and Kim West, MSW

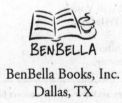

BenBella Books, Inc.
Dallas, TX

BenBella Books, Inc.
10440 N. Central Expressway
Suite 800
Dallas, TX 75231
benbellabooks.com
Send feedback to feedback@benbellabooks.com

BenBella is a federally registered trademark.

Printed in the United States of America
10 9 8 7 6 5 4 3 2 1

Library of Congress Control Number: 2024022706
ISBN 9781637745335 (trade paperback)
ISBN 9781637745342 (electronic)

Editing by Leah Wilson
Copyediting by Jessica Easto
Proofreading by Lisa Story and Sarah Vostok
Text design and composition by PerfecType
Cover design by Morgan Carr
Cover image © iStock / Juanmonino
Printed by Lake Book Manufacturing

Special discounts for bulk sales are available. Please contact bulkorders@benbellabooks.com.

To Gretchen, my livewire daughter who has taught me to read and respond differently as a mother and has helped me to be a better Sleep Lady. And to all the parents of livewires who I have helped over the last 30 years who have opened their hearts to me and who I continue to learn from. You, too, have helped me to be a better Sleep Lady. Thank you with all my heart! And finally, Macall, who has inadvertently guided me to see more clearly the sensitive livewire in me.

—Kim

To my two livewires, Madison and Jake, who set me on this path, pushed me, and filled me up with joy; and to my husband Jonathan (also a livewire) who has been with me on this journey of parenting while figuring out our own temperaments.

And to all the parents of livewires, who, even when they feel like nothing is working and they are so tired they might just collapse, still get up every day and strive to be the best that they can be for their brilliant, blazing handful of a child. This book is for you.

—Macall

CONTENTS

INTRODUCTION

Mention sleep training in just about any online parenting discussion, and it's like you've just lit a fuse and started the countdown. I've seen *so many* comment threads get shut down because it gets *so hot so fast*. Rather than an exchange of ideas, it quickly becomes a war between two sides lobbing judgment bombs at each other. One side says that parents set the rules and crying it out is both effective and a small price to pay for better sleep. The other side thinks that crying it out in any context is harmful, and parents should follow their baby's cues. Both sides are certain that their approach is the most effective and appropriate for babies . . . because, for their child, it *worked*.

You know who's *not* in this fight? *Everyone else*. These are the parents who are exhausted, bewildered, and desperate because *nothing* has worked, despite trying a whole smorgasbord of strategies. While the sleep wars rage on, these parents are hanging on by their fingernails, left to wonder what they are doing wrong and whether they will ever sleep again.

This was definitely me. My first one had her eyes wide open right from the get-go. She never, ever slept, and even at two months, she acted like sleeping was a waste of precious time. Trying to get a nap was a marathon of bouncing furiously on a yoga ball just to get twenty minutes of shut-eye. My son, on the other hand, was a decent napper and would fall asleep quickly at bedtime, but he would wake every forty-five minutes all night.

Each of them had a different but still ridiculously challenging sleep pattern. Nighttime never went anything like the experts said it would.

Back then, there were three options for working on sleep: cry it out, co-sleep, or wait it out. I knew that if I were even able to attempt crying it out, my stunning and persistent babies would cry like they were dying for *hours* and never give up ever, ever. So, instead, I leaned into the advice to follow their cues, since the experts said that *that* would lead to better sleep. Nope. Even co-sleeping wasn't working. I was left with just waiting until it got better. Rock, meet hard place.

Today, not a lot has changed. Sleep advice is everywhere, but it's almost always suggesting some version of leaving the room, with the same promise of sleeping through the night in three to seven days. For some parents, that *is* what happens. But for lots of other parents . . . not so much. Even in research studies, cry it out didn't work for between 20 and 40 percent of families. But parents don't get to hear that little truth nugget. As a result, they're left thinking that maybe they're just no good at this parenting thing.

Nope. Not true.

We know that temperament plays a clear role in sleep behavior. Research has found that a "difficult" temperament—intense, difficult to soothe, etc.—is a big predictor of sleep problems[1] and that young children with this temperament do not respond as well or as fast to cry it out as more easygoing children do.[2] However, *none* of the research on sleep training has taken temperament into account. We know nothing about how more intense, sensitive children respond to cry it out approaches. Is it possible that a big chunk of those 20 to 40 percent were actually children who had a "difficult" temperament? Is it possible that cry it out doesn't work that well for this whole group of children? (Spoiler alert: Yes, it's totally possible. But no one has asked that question yet.)

As a researcher, I've gathered a lot of data from parents about temperament and sleep. I surveyed 850 parents of children ages six months to six years to find out about the relationship between temperament and sleep. The results showed that children who were intense, sensitive, and alert had significantly more trouble with *every* aspect of sleep (not a shock) and that their parents had tried a higher number of sleep methods with much less success than parents of mellower children.

I had also noticed that nearly all the research on children's temperament focused on those "difficult" traits and their risk factors and long-term negative outcomes. Given my experience with my own children, I knew there was a lot more in that temperament package than just the "difficult" stuff. My kiddos *were* rough sleepers, but they were also bright and outspoken and persistent and perceptive. I decided to test whether other children who would be labeled as "difficult" by researchers had positive traits that no one had thought to look for. My survey results found that the children who had higher levels of challenging traits also had higher levels of some positive ones—like perceptiveness, empathy, sense of fairness, and persistence.

You have picked up this book, so Kim and I are guessing that there's not much sleep going on in your house and you might be struggling to get the little bit you *are* getting. We're also guessing that you have a child with some of the following traits: alert, engaged, curious, intense, perceptive, persistent, and smarter than they should be for their age. Every one of those traits (and more that we'll talk about) contributes to a child having more trouble getting to sleep and staying asleep. Understanding what specific traits make sleep difficult is game changing because it means that you can finally work on sleep with this information in mind. It's not easy—I'm not going to lie—but the work will be worth it to get you out of whatever Rube Goldberg sleep contraption you're in now.

We are going to spend the following chapters talking about your unique child. We are going to discover, together, who they are, what makes sleep so difficult for them to achieve, and what you will need to do to finally get more of it. We're going to talk about the challenges of temperament, as well as the incredible silver-lining qualities that come with it. Then, we'll craft a plan for edging them toward more manageable sleep patterns. And the best news of all? This process does not require you to leave your little one alone in a room to cry. You will not have to set a timer or "steel yourself."

We are going to proceed gradually, giving a lot of support at first, and we're going to do everything possible to make sure that this process is tolerable for *everyone* (sensitive adults included).

This isn't going to be a walk in the park. You have a bigger hill to climb than friends (potentially all of them) who have an "easier" child. However, if you are prepared for it—if you have the right map, the right equipment, and a few dozen protein bars in your backpack—it's totally doable. We've taken a lot of parents on this trek, and when you use tools that actually fit *your child*, it really, really works.

TEAMING UP WITH KIM WEST, MSW (AKA THE SLEEP LADY)

Before I became a sleep coach, and about ten years after I became a mom, I enrolled in a graduate psychology program to really dive into the question of whether the sleep training advice I had been reading all those years was supported by research. (Spoiler alert: It wasn't.) I studied infant mental health, attachment, emotional regulation, research methods, and family systems to better understand sleep, parenting, and the world of parenting advice. After receiving my master's degree and teaching therapists-in-training for a number of years, I realized that maybe it was time to take what I knew and what I had learned and use it to actually help parents with sleep.

In 2015, I began looking for a training program that took a systemic approach to sleep. The deal-breaker was that it had to offer an alternative to cry it out. That's when I met Kim. Her training program was rigorous, multidisciplinary, and offered a balanced way to look at sleep—both from the child's point of view and the parents'. It just made a lot of sense.

She not only had a background in mental health but had also raised a child like mine. Kim's first child was fairly easygoing. Her second, however, not so much. This one was born three weeks early and had horrible eczema and silent reflux that took two months to diagnose and multiple medications to get under control. Once her baby was finally no longer in pain, Kim was finally able to get her to sleep, but only in very specific conditions. Everything had to be just so—dark room, her own crib. Even after the reflux resolved, Kim's little force of nature continued to be very sensory sensitive and persnickety, and she went from zero to a hundred in seconds flat—full-on fling-yourself-on-the-ground-and-bang-your-head meltdowns.

We had both tried to parent our alert little ones with the books and magazines available at the time (mercifully, the internet was just barely a thing) and were left feeling like those experts were just not talking about our children. Needless to say, we had *a lot* of common experiences with and perspectives on sleep and sleep training. Kim and I were in the same boat as new moms—knowing that Ferber was not the answer for our baby fireballs. I just kept following my children's nonexistent "sleepy cues" until I hit a brick wall. Kim, on the other hand, had the presence of mind to know there must be a better way. (Boy, do I wish we had known each other back then.)

With her first, she had crafted a gradual, methodical, totally common-sense approach to sleep training that wasn't just Ferber with a different name. She offered a lot of support, presence, and calming and then gradually reduced it over time as her child learned how to sleep on her own. What was to become the Sleep Lady Shuffle had really worked for her first (mostly easygoing) little one. She used this method with her second (alert, sensitive) baby, too, and again it really worked. When it also worked for the families she coached, she knew she was onto something.

Across the more than twenty thousand families she has successfully helped using the Shuffle, Kim estimates that as many as 75 percent of them had a child she recognized as having an alert temperament. And she found that the Shuffle consistently worked when other methods, like cry it out, had not. I have also found this to be true for the thousands of families in my own practice, where I specialize in these alert, non-sleeping little ones.

I'm sure you already have figured out that fixing sleep is more than knowing what steps to take. It's the execution of those steps—especially with a child that just doesn't fit the "typical" mold. The way *you* approach sleep needs to be different because you do not have an easy, go-with-the-flow child. We'll use Kim's gradual, responsive approach in this book, but we'll also help you understand all the moving parts involved in getting better sleep and why other methods just haven't worked for you.

Possibly the biggest reason for a more specialized focus, however, is that you have unique needs as a *parent* of an alert little one. You may be the only parent you know who has a child like yours. You may have felt for a while now that no one else really understands what you are going through. That stops now.

We hope this book lets you know that you are definitely not alone. There are so many parents like you stuck in the middle of the sleep wars, feeling like maybe they're just not good at this whole parenting thing. We're going to change that. Your child isn't struggling with sleep because you're "doing it wrong." You aren't causing it, and you're not overreacting. Your problems are bigger, the pushback is stronger, and the expert advice wasn't written about *your* child. We're going to change that last thing, too. We're going to speak directly to *your* experiences. Parents who've seen the material in this book tell us that they finally feel *seen*. We want that to be true for you, too. In addition to solid information about development, temperament, and sleep, a fair bit of this book is devoted to *you* and making sure you have what you need to steer this big sleep (and life) bus like the rock star you are.

Doesn't that sound awesome?

SECTION ONE

You Are Here: Getting the Lay of the Land

CHAPTER 1

So, Every Sleep Training Method So Far Has Been an Epic Fail

If you have honestly tried every sleep method out there—Ferber, pop-ins, the Sleep Fairy, cold turkey, co-sleeping, melatonin, praying that it magically just gets better—and nothing (I mean, *nothing*) has worked, I have good news for you: Your lack of success has nothing to do with what you have or haven't done. The big reason that sleep training methods haven't worked so far has to do with *your child's temperament*—the way they are innately wired. Children who easily get with the program after a couple of nights of tolerable struggle or gentle encouragement are simply more easygoing and adjust to changes in familiar patterns without a lot of drama. I'm betting you don't have one of those children. You, dear pooped-out parent, probably have what I call a *livewire*.

WHAT IN THE WORLD IS A LIVEWIRE?

Livewires are children who have more physical, mental, and emotional juice flowing through their system. They are deeply feeling, highly sensitive, keenly perceptive, incredibly engaged, insanely persistent, ridiculously smart, super active, interaction-addicted supernovas. Kim, in her work, refers to these little ones as "alert" . . . and boy, are they.

As a result:

- "Drowsy but awake" never has been and *never will* be in their vocabulary.
- Resisting sleep is their full-time job.
- They can go from calm to screaming faster than you can say "pacifier."
- They are not "self-soothers."
- They can be sound asleep, and the slightest noise will still make their eyes *pop* open.

A livewire temperament means that sleep training using the popular methods *isn't* a matter of a few challenging nights of tolerable crying. That first night was probably more like two straight hours of crying with no sign that your child was *ever* going to give in and go to sleep. Or maybe you never attempted it in the first place because you already knew it was a nonstarter. Instead, you've cobbled together something that barely kind of works but is completely unsustainable. I'm betting you're wondering why sleep training is so impossible for you. I'm also betting that you are exhausted, burned out, and more sleep-deprived than a human should be. You are not the only one.

Both Kim and I have worked with *a lot* of parents who needed help with sleep. Not because they'd never tried to fix things. No. They needed help because they had tried *every bit* of advice they'd gotten from books or their pediatrician or Instagram or their friends, and *none of it* worked. Nearly all these desperate parents had an alert little livewire.

Have you ever made any of these statements about your child?

"They go from zero to screaming bloody murder if I don't respond quickly."
"We spend hours bouncing on the ball to get them to sleep."

"Once they get really upset, it's hard to calm them down."

"They hate (H-A-T-E) the car seat (or swaddle)."

"They just do not want to sleep. It's like they're afraid they'll miss something."

"They're either asleep or go, go, go like the Energizer Bunny. There's no in-between."

"We can get them dead asleep, and the minute we lay them down, their eyes pop open, and we have to start all over."

"They're my Sour Patch Kid—super sassy and sour but also just the sweetest."

Does any of this sound familiar? If you're thinking, *That's my child . . .*

You, my friend, have a livewire.

Parents often know something is up right from the beginning or soon after. *"Is it possible for a newborn to fight sleep?"* *"How is it my two-month-old seems bored?"*

Did your little one express any of these traits right out of the gate?

Very early alertness (eyes *wide* open and focused just after birth)

Really vigorous crying (Did the nurses comment about it in the hospital? *"This one is going to be a handful."* *"They've got some lungs on them."*)

Totally sleep-avoidant, even as a newborn

Visually engaged (loved looking at faces, pictures, etc.)

Able to hold head up early

Preference for being bounced to sleep (versus rocked)

Livewires are just different from other children. I don't have to tell you this; you are likely already living it. They're fussier / more emotional. They walk or talk much earlier. They sleep so much less. There are so many ways that these little ones diverge from what you might have expected or seen before. It's normal to wonder why your child (and your experience as a parent) is so different from the others.

IF YOU'VE ALREADY TRIED SEVERAL METHODS WITH YOUR (OVER SIX-MONTH-OLD) LIVEWIRE WITH ZERO SUCCESS . . . IT'S NOT YOUR FAULT

Authors of the most popular sleep books will say that if you follow their "easy" steps, you can lay your baby in the crib, leave the room, and barely hear a peep all night. They say that if you just leave your child alone to figure things out, they will learn to go to sleep without help in just a few days.

Here's a big secret you should know:

99 percent of sleep books are not written about livewires.

In fact, they don't even consider temperament as a factor.

Most children (non-livewires) will, with a little nudging or even a few nights of tolerable distress, get on board with a new routine. Their path to sleep is clear and well marked, and they don't have that far to go. For these children, parents *can* mostly stay out of the way because it's not that hard for the child to figure out how to get from point A (awake) to point B (asleep). For livewires, the trail to sleep is *not* smooth, short, or well marked; it is steeper and rockier, and the destination seems a lot farther away. Livewires need a map, a GPS, and a couple of sherpas to help them get to sleep.

Trying to use methods that have been devised for non-livewires on your livewire child is like trying to use the manual for the wrong computer. You can read a Mac manual all day long, but if you have a PC, those instructions will not be helpful at all. What may be straightforward, effective, and doable for other parents is just not going to work the same way for you.

For less intense children, it's possible that just about *anything* will work. It's the opposite if you have a livewire. *Nothing* works like the books or internet (or other parents) say it will. I remember reading parenting magazines about sleep training that made it sound *so simple*: "Make sure to put your baby down when they're still awake so they can fall asleep on their own."

Okay, here we go. Aaand cue head-spinning hysterics. *Okay, sleep expert, what am I supposed to do <u>now</u>?*

There was not one more word about it, like sleep was just supposed to— *poof*—happen. I constantly worried that I was doing something wrong. *If there were more to it, if it were potentially more of a challenge, they would have said something, right?* But the experts *didn't* say anything, and I was left with a non-sleeping livewire and a nagging worry that maybe I wasn't cut out for any of this.

Chances are, you've had well-meaning friends or family members tell you, "Oh, I tried the XYZ method, and in just a few nights, the baby was totally sleeping through! You should try that!" or "You just have to suck it up and let them cry it out. You're too soft." (How often have you heard *that* one?)

Let's take it as a given that you have worked sleep up one side and down the other. If the straightforward behavioral advice had worked, you wouldn't be reading this book.

THE DREADED "ARE THEY SLEEPING THROUGH THE NIGHT?"

Having a "good sleeper" has become a kind of crazy benchmark of parenting skill. It's nuts. Everyone seems to have *that* friend who says that her three-month-old is sleeping six to eight hours straight without a feed, and it's because she used that "great new method . . . that *you* should try." At three months, I can promise you—that baby's considerable ability to sleep had nothing to do with what their parents did (or did not do). The baby was wired for sleep. But because we mistakenly tell parents that sleep is exclusively about *behavior* (what parents do or don't do) and that babies *can* and *must* be trained to sleep, parents of good sleepers can be led to believe it was because of them. The truth is that this process is way easier for many babies and next to impossible for others—simply because of temperament.

> **The dividing line between children who sleep and those who don't isn't the sleep method you use—it's temperament.**

This situation is not helped by the tone of advice that can make you feel like your child's future hinges on whether or not they are a "good sleeper." Parents are strongly warned that poor sleep affects brain development and can cause obesity, ADHD, behavioral problems, and a whole host of other worrying outcomes. (And just so you don't panic, sleep problems do not *cause* those outcomes. Just because two things are related in some way doesn't mean that one *caused* the other.) It's no wonder parents are tied up in knots about how to get their babies sleeping for long periods of time as early as possible.

Sleep advice in general is full of parent-shaming and gaslighting. If you try their version of cry it out, your baby cries for *hours*, and you finally respond because you can't bear it anymore, you are "caving," "weak," or "permissive." Believe it or not, in medical journals, there is now a diagnosis under "infant sleep disorders" called *limit-setting disorder* . . . and they're not talking about the baby. Reluctance to begin or complete sleep training is now a disorder? Bonkers.

When we focus exclusively on behavior—what parents *do* or *don't* do in response to crying—then the blame falls on the parent if it doesn't work. But "Just try harder" should not be the only response to "This isn't working." There are so many factors that can influence a child's sleep, and we're going to be looking at the big picture—*everything* that influences sleep: development, physiology, temperament, your bandwidth, and your preferences or needs (you want to continue co-sleeping, you don't have another room for the baby, etc.). With children as complex as livewires, a simple one-size-fits-all approach isn't going to cut it. We need to address all the moving parts—starting with the big one that sets the tone: temperament.

WHAT DOES TEMPERAMENT HAVE TO DO WITH SLEEP? EVERYTHING.

It's surprising that sleep research and advice don't consider temperament more than they do, since just about everything related to the process of going to sleep and staying asleep is directly affected by it. *Temperament* refers to the hardwired neurological system we use to monitor and process input from the outside world. For most children (non-livewires), this system can detect some input and buffer out the rest. About 20 percent of children (though I believe this is a low estimate)—livewires—have an internal system that is *much* more sensitive to input (they pick up on a lot more) and that reacts much more strongly to that input. Basically, it takes less input to get a stronger reaction.

This hardwiring isn't theoretical. Biologists have found that there are genetic components to the sensitivity we see in livewires and that children can be roughly divided into two types: *dandelions* (non-livewires) and *orchids* (livewires).[3] Dandelions, as plants, grow pretty darned well in a wide variety of environments. They can thrive almost anywhere (really— *anywhere*). Most children are dandelions, wired to adapt to a wide variety of environments. Their internal fight-or-flight systems are not easily alerted, and they are able to thrive even under some stress or adversity. They do pretty well in a very wide range of contexts, and they are fairly resilient in the face of negative events.

A much smaller group of children are orchids. If you've ever tried to grow an orchid, you know that they need a *very* specific set of circumstances to really flourish. Outside of this tiny niche of *just* the right amount of light, humidity, and water, they can fizzle. Children who have orchid-type wiring (livewires) are genetically more reactive and sensitive to their environment. They are much more likely to struggle in the face of much smaller challenges and disruptions.

This means that two children—one an orchid and one a dandelion—who experience the same event will respond very differently. The dandelion may be able to buffer out the stress of it and recover fairly well. The orchid, on the other hand, may be much more deeply affected and will have a much harder time bouncing back. The big research term for this is *differential susceptibility to environment.*[4]

Here's some really good news: The flip side of an orchid's strong reaction to *negative* experiences is that they also respond more strongly to *positive* ones. While it's true that orchids need master gardener–level care and handling, if they get it, they really, really bloom. Researchers Michael Pluess and Jay Belsky call this *vantage sensitivity.*[5] While dandelion children do equally well in a variety of environments, orchid children are more vulnerable to negative events or environments *and* benefit even *more* from positive ones.

This notion that strengths and challenges are a package deal is going to be an ongoing theme of this book. Orchids require a ton of work, but they produce amazing flowers. Same with livewires. You may have an incredibly fussy, non-sleeping baby who is also incredibly social and verbal. You may have a toddler who comes up with every reason in the book for why they can't go to sleep at bedtime who is also hilariously funny and creative and can name every species of dinosaur. Pluess and Belsky call these strengths the "bright sides" of temperament.[6] Their perspective (and mine too) is that research is overly focused on the difficult sides of a more intense temperament and overlooks the significant abilities that go along with it. My research on temperament bright sides shows that, sure enough, while a more intense, sensitive temperament was related to *tons* of sleep problems (like *all* of them), there were also impressive strengths in that package, like empathy, perceptiveness, and engagement.

Parents don't need research to tell them this. They already know. Talk to any livewire parent, and they will tell you that, yes, they are about to fall over from fatigue, but their little one is "so social," "early on their milestones," and "knows more than they should be able to at this age." As Kim says, "It was like Gretchen had an adult soul in a tiny body." Having a livewire is both incredibly challenging and completely amazing.

If you have been really struggling for a while, it may feel like you're living full-time in the hard, dark side of temperament. It may be difficult to detect even the *possibility* that a bright side exists. I know that feeling. There can be long stretches where the upsides are hard to detect. I promise the silver linings are there. They really are. They just masquerade as a lot of unsettled crying and upset at first, before your livewire develops the capacity to drive their brain. It's like putting a new driver in a Ferrari. They just don't have the skill to manage that amount of horsepower . . . yet. Eventually, they will. And then stand back. They are going to really take off.

PARENTING A LIVEWIRE IS A WHOLE DIFFERENT BALL GAME

If you have a livewire, you are on a path that's different from most, or even all, of your peers. How often have you already wondered what other parents are doing to have a child who plays contentedly in their high chair or who can sit in a carrier while their mom gets her hair cut? It's incredibly important for us to acknowledge and validate that your road as a parent is harder, and you've probably second-guessed yourself a million times. Making sure that *you* are seen and that your struggles are understood in this process is key.

Kim and I, combined, have worked with tens of thousands of parents of livewires who have shared surprisingly similar experiences and concerns. See if any of these sound familiar.

"This is not at all like I thought it would be."

This one is a biggie. Parents who have livewires often know right out of the gate that they're not in Kansas anymore. It's not uncommon for them to report a long, difficult, or even traumatic labor and/or birth. (We don't know why this is, but my survey also found this relationship.) If, after that, you also had a really unsettled, nonsleeping newborn, you might already be wondering what you have signed up for. This is no Pampers ad.

Having a livewire can throw you off your center as a parent because the reality is so drastically different from what we expected or were told to expect. It's not at all helped by others around you who think there's an obvious, no-brainer reason why your baby acts this way.

"He cries so much because you just keep picking him up."

"Have you tried gas drops?"

Then, there's the advice from books or your pediatrician that you should "just" . . . well, anything.

"Just swaddle her."

"Just let him cry a little, and he'll learn."

Or the one that really gets me, *"It's just colic."*

If you have a newborn who isn't sleeping and is screaming for most of the day, you know that saying *"It's just colic"* is like saying *"It's just a tidal wave."* We are not talking about the normal and expected levels of fussiness. Livewires tend to be at least one notch (or ten) above "normal." For many parents, when their baby cries and they respond, the baby is soothed, and the parent gets the message, *I know my baby. I think I know what I'm doing.* When you have a newborn livewire, on the other hand, you don't get many moments of *I've got this.* This bumpy start can be the first step in a long road of feeling like you have no idea what you're doing. If you had this really, really difficult start or are still in the midst of it—know you are a warrior, and you've got this more than you think you do.

"There's so . . . much . . . crying." (Your baby, but also you.)

Livewires can express themselves much, much more intensely and urgently than other babies. My newborn daughter never "fussed." When she cried, it was like she had been stuck with a pin—it was intense and urgent. I remember almost panicking and thinking, *Do I need to take her to the emergency room?* One mom on Facebook admitted: "I would hear other babies' cute, sweet 'cries,' while my daughter's regular normal cry sounded like her limbs were being ripped off her body."

The inconsolable nature of the crying is something that's particularly hard on new parents. Some researchers suggest that, evolutionarily, these babies would have done really well. As hunter-gatherer newborns, these squeaky wheels would have received a lot of extra parental attention, closeness, and care. Livewires demand a higher level of parenting investment and effort.[7] And the good news, wiped-out mamas, papas, and others? You are ponying up. Well done, you.

"I'm beyond exhausted."

Across the dandelion–orchid spectrum, all parents are pooped. As a parent of a livewire, you are guaranteed to be emotionally and physically *beyond* pooped. Sleep problems can be intense and, almost always, have been around practically from birth. Additionally, livewires don't just struggle at night; they require more from parents during the day, too. Oh, boy. "Tired" doesn't even describe it.

It's important to know that this book is going to take your level of exhaustion into account. You won't be able to make this journey if you are completely out of gas. Together, we'll figure out a plan for getting where you want to go even if you're running on fumes.

"My child isn't like the other children I know (or even like the other children I have)."

If this livewire is your first child, you may have doubted your own assessment: *Is my baby actually different from other children? Or am I just totally out of it? How do I even know?* It's easy to feel like the odd duck in a group of other parents and children. Yours seems to be the only child that gets so upset or can't calm down. They always seem to need special handling. Livewires just don't inhabit the world in the same way as other children. I remember talking to a neighbor who had her eight-month-old sitting in a pram next to us. She gave the baby an empty plastic water bottle to play with, and that baby played with it for *a full forty-five minutes*. I kept staring and wondering what kind of strange magic this was. If it had been either of my children, that bottle would have been tossed out of the pram in fifteen seconds flat ("Done with that. Next?"). I hear parents of livewires admit a certain amount of envy of parents with easier kids. This is normal and understandable. "Easier" can look pretty good. But remember, your live-wire is an orchid. The payoffs from the time and energy you put into them may be farther down the road—but I promise you, they're there.

"It's just a lot."

Livewires require more from their parents around the clock. Even when they're happy, they want and need lots of engagement and interaction. There are so many questions and stories and thoughts and ideas. When they're not happy or when they're tired, it's a different kind of rodeo. Add to this the amount of worry and struggle you may have around sleep, and it's hard on the nervous system. You may be at a point where you will do just about *anything* to have less crying and conflict. You have probably given in on so many limits or done what's "easy" just to stop the crying for one brief moment. I get it. I've been there. It's okay. We're going to start from wherever you are now and work to get a leg up on sleep.

"I worry that I just suck at parenting."

This is one of the *most important* messages of this book:

You do not suck at parenting.

Single, divorced, stay at home, full-time job with childcare, work at home—whatever your situation, you are a rock star. You may not feel it. You may not believe me. You may not be able to see evidence of it in your daily life. But I promise you, you are a dedicated, roll-up-your-sleeves, in-for-the-long-haul parent. Livewires don't give you the same in-the-moment confirmation that what you just did actually worked, the way other children might. You mostly have to go on blind faith, which can feel discouraging. It's hard to see the proof that you're making good choices, but you are.

Struggles with sleep may be at the very heart of these feelings of suckiness. Most parents of livewires have tried several gadgets, programs, and "guaranteed" methods to get better sleep. We wouldn't blame you if you were skeptical about whether *anything* will work. Plus, you've seen too many books that promise an effective, gentle approach only to trot out the same old *"You have to leave the room, or they'll never learn to self-soothe."* I am happy to say that we are going to take a different approach.

HOW THIS PROCESS WILL BE DIFFERENT FROM THE OTHER METHODS YOU'VE TRIED

You already know that the road to better sleep is not simple or straightforward. And the way we're going to approach it will be different from much of what you have already tried. This is why we use the term *sleep coaching* instead of *sleep training*: It's not about "habits" that need to be "broken." We're going to be helping and encouraging new patterns. We are also going to help you understand *all* the moving parts involved in making sleep happen so that you can make choices that will work for you and your unique livewire. We're going to validate and acknowledge *you* and the boatloads of effort you put into your parenting. We're going to understand your livewire's specific temperament traits and how those are affecting their sleep (and your attempt to get more). We're going to rule out anything that could be getting in the way of sleep. And we're going to break the process into manageable pieces. Most importantly:

We're not going to have anyone crying by themselves in a room (you or your livewire).

WHAT YOU SHOULD KNOW
BEFORE WE DIVE IN

Chances are, you're coming to this work already battle-scarred, probably exhausted, and feeling defeated. We can't let you start from there. Here's some validation and reassurance, and a little straight talk before we take the plunge.

The crazy stuff you have had to do up to this point to get sleep is okay.

In the absence of having anything that *actually worked*, you may have had to cobble together something resembling a strategy from snippets of what *did* work, at least temporarily. Parents who have resorted to nontraditional shenanigans to get their child to sleep are often carrying a truckload of shame around it.

I hear it from parents all the time:

"I know I've probably encouraged a lot of bad habits."
"I know that was probably a bad decision, but we just had to sleep."
"I've probably really screwed things up by doing this, but . . ."
"I know it's bad, but we have to co-sleep / nurse all night / sleep in their room . . ."

If you feel like you have made really "out there" choices in the service of sleep, you are not alone. In addition to all the nursing and rocking and lying in a toddler bed and driving around for hours, you probably had to reach for any shred of traction you could get.

Here are just a few of the "extra" strategies I've heard from parents:

Walking on a treadmill while carrying the baby
Letting the child fall asleep with their finger in the parent's mouth or playing with the parent's eyebrow
Running (not walking) outside with the baby

Lying on the floor out of view while jingling a set of bells

Getting in the crib with the baby

Doing squats with the baby while singing or humming "Jingle Bells"

Singing "Stand by Me" while bouncing on a yoga ball and with a hand vacuum running on the floor (this was me)

Letting the child fall asleep on the parent's arm and then carefully extracting it once asleep (the child, and possibly the arm)

Almost violent bouncing on an exercise ball

Turning on the dryer and the vacuum and rolling the vacuum back and forth while bouncing the baby over a shoulder and singing a particular pop song

Having to perform this level of gymnastics to get your child to power down can add an extra layer of "I suck" on top of the sleep troubles you already have. I am giving you permission to ditch that now. Whatever parenting gymnastics you've had to perform to get sleep up to this point made sense in the sleep-deprived, desperate moment you were in. Maybe some of it even worked—at least for a bit. Do not feel bad for what you tried or for how you got here. Offload the guilt. You were responding to the child you have, and you needed to do *something*. Now, we are going to figure out a different way that will make sense for your unique livewire. Keep reading.

We're not going to sugarcoat it.

We're not going to use terms like *sweet sleep* or *peaceful slumber* or *a little bit of protest*. Nope. We're going to call it like it is. We are not going to be afraid to say how insanely hard this can be. We'll be honest about the fact that it's going to get worse before it gets better.

Wait, what? Worse? I can't do worse.

I hear you. It's okay. Take a breath. We've got you.

We're also not going to gloss over the fact that parenting an intense / sensitive livewire can get dark more often than we'd like: eruptions of rage, massive desperation, feelings of wanting to run away. Parents often

judge themselves for those feelings. But when you are pushed to the edges
of your stamina, there can be monsters in that closet. We're going to look
those beasts right in the eye. Having a livewire is never what you expect.
It can come as a full-frontal assault to every expectation you have. Sweet
moments sitting in the rocking chair? Nope. Lunch with friends while the
baby naps in the stroller? Nope. Feelings of calm contentedness while your
baby coos happily on their play mat? Nope, nope, nope. The reality of parenting one of these tornados can be a desperate, sweaty, dirty, tearstained
affair. I remember all that bubble bath nonsense you'd hear and see on TV:
"A bubble bath can be great self-care." Me: *"But I just have to come back to
my life once I get out!"* (dissolves in sobs). As parents, we have to (and do)
hold both: Our kids are bright, incredible, amazing creatures, and we're so
overwhelmed, we just might collapse.

We're going to base what we say in research (but with a little bit of side-eye).

Research is a powerful tool, but not all research is our friend. There are
many, many ways that research can ignore critical pieces of information or
can be set up in ways that work for research but don't map at all to real life.
It can also be (shocker) biased. We will refer to research but will not hesitate
to call it out on its shenanigans.

You are not a parenting Pez dispenser.

Sleep and parenting advice consistently make it sound as if you are just a
passive dispenser of parenting strategies. I remember reading about positive
parenting strategies, trying to use them in a tough moment, and thinking,
*How am I supposed to be "positive" when I feel like I'm about to jump out of
my skin?* Whatever parenting we do is absolutely filtered through our own
temperament and experiences, and it's powered by how much energy we
have in the moment—which I'm betting is not usually a heckuva lot.

In working on sleep, we *have to* take your bandwidth into account. Having to confront a lot of around-the-clock intensity (meltdowns, tantrums, cranky-pants screaming) can cause you to be—honestly—a little shell-shocked. I know you sometimes would seriously do *anything* to make it stop. I get that, and it makes sense. By the time many parents find their way to me, their stamina and energy stores have been ground down to a powder. They literally can't tolerate the situation getting even a tiny bit worse. While it's better when parents reach out *before* they're rock-bottom adjacent, if you feel like that right now, it's okay. I will show you how to break sleep and temperament down into actionable steps that feel doable. The goal is to work on sleep in ways that don't blow you (or your child) out of the water.

We're going to wait to work on sleep until babies are at least six months old.

If you have a younger little one, don't freak out. There is good information in this book that will be useful to you both now and moving forward. We know that there's a lot of information out there that says you can (and should) start training newborns to sleep for long periods of time and that if you don't start early, it will be harder.

First, please don't worry about sleep training your newborn. There's no research on the safety or effectiveness of sleep training at this age and very little on using cry it out on babies under six months. In this first half of infancy, there is a lot of critical brain and nervous system development that has to happen, and trying to establish patterns or letting them cry to "help them learn" doesn't make any sense. A newborn has none of the skills or coordination necessary for managing their sleep. So, we wait until they do.

There's a lot more on this point in chapter four. (If you want some non-sleep-training strategies to improve sleep for younger babies, however, you can check out *The Sleep Lady's Gentle Newborn Sleep Guide*.)

This isn't a cry it out approach (and it isn't completely "no cry," either).

Real talk? There is no way to change a livewire's sleep patterns in ways they won't notice. They *will* notice and then they will let us know that they notice. While it's possible to do some of the steps in smaller pieces or at a slower pace, when children are this aware and perceptive, the change you make would have to be microscopically small for it to fly under their radar.

That said . . . here are a few promises we will make to you:

- We're not going to talk you into leaving your child alone to figure things out without help.
- We're not going to place any value on crying as a "learning experience."
- We're going to do everything possible to set everyone up for success and minimize distress.
- We are going to scaffold skills gradually and offer your livewire a lot of presence and support at first.
- We are not going to let them get hysterical and then say they've learned something when they finally fall asleep.
- We're going to make sure that you feel as good as possible about the strategies you use (because, spoiler alert, you'll probably have to use them again at some point).

Sleep is just one small part of the larger experience.

More real talk here: Your parenting challenges are not going to disappear once sleep is handled. The road with a livewire does not magically become flat and smooth once they are sleeping. *You* will feel like a whole new person once you get some sleep, and your child might be a little less frazzled. But they will still be the same active, alert, sensitive livewire they were before. The great news is that the concepts we cover in our work on sleep (predictability, consistency, support) will also come in super handy in the long-term.

WHAT YOU WILL NEED FOR THE ROAD AHEAD

So, with all of that in mind, we're going to set aside what you may have already read about sleep. That information and those strategies work for parents on a totally different (flatter, shorter, more well-marked) path. You are not on that path. Though the destination is the same, your path is longer, steeper, and rockier (but with some amazing views from the top).

In the coming chapters, we are going to get you loaded up with everything you will need to take on this journey. We're going to do a lot of preparation before you even hit the road. We're going to check to make sure your child is ready and that *you* are ready. We're going to ensure you know what the terrain looks like and what the potential road hazards are along the way. Then, we are going to give you the right map and the right equipment to help you get to your destination in a way that makes sense and is tolerable for both you *and* your livewire. We're also going to give you a set of tools to assess whether you're off course and, if so, how to get back on track. We're going to go step by step.

To this end, we've created a set of downloadable worksheets that will help you better understand where you are now and the best way to get where you want to go. As we move through the material, watch for the callouts about which sheet to use for each section.

WORKBOOK TO DO

Download the Workbook by going to whywontyousleep.com/workbook or scanning the QR code:

So take a breath, relax your shoulders. We've taken lots of parents up this mountain. Ready to go?

OUR TRIP CHECKLIST

- ☑ **You know you are on a different path.**
- ☐ You understand your livewire's temperament strengths and challenges.
- ☐ You understand the link between temperament and sleep issues.
- ☐ Your child is ready:
  - ☐ Over six months
  - ☐ No upcoming disruptions
  - ☐ No physiological issues that affect sleep
- ☐ You are ready (or as ready as you can be).
- ☐ You understand the Big Four sources of sleep issues.
- ☐ Big Strategy #1: You know how to avoid that second wind.
- ☐ Big Strategy #2: You have a solid, consistent bedtime routine.
- ☐ Big Strategy #3 and #4: You know how to change the go-to-sleep and back-to-sleep patterns and are prepared to be more consistent than you've ever been before.
- ☐ You know how to track progress.
- ☐ You know how to diagnose and fix any problems that arise.
- ☐ BETTER SLEEP!

CHAPTER 2

Assessing the Terrain: Mapping Livewire Temperament

Before we can dive into solving your tricky sleep issues, we first need to know how your little livewire is wired. What are their challenges? What are their strengths? And how do both of those impact sleep and your attempts to get more of it for everyone? Without a solid understanding of what your child is bringing to the table in terms of temperament, all the sleep advice in the world won't make a bit of difference. Before we can start on that trek to better sleep, we need to know what lies ahead in terms of the terrain. Understanding temperament is the key to all of that.

CRACKING THE TEMPERAMENT CODE

Children come into the world with biologically determined wiring that dictates how they will detect, receive, and process input from the internal and external world. Think about satellite dishes. Some huge ones are designed to track the movements of satellites, comets, planets, and stars. Some are smaller and focus on picking up and transmitting only your streaming service and nothing else. Imagine babies as being born with a similar kind of internal satellite dish. To some, lights and sounds and texture and temperature hit their receptors all at once as superstrong signals that easily overload their developing circuitry. Other babies, ones with detection systems focused only on a few of those incoming signals, are able to buffer out the rest.

Parents with more than one child often see firsthand how stark the differences can be in two children's wiring. Baby 1 struggles with just about everything: almost never sleeps, maybe has or had colic or reflux or eczema, and needs tons of input and soothing. But Baby 2 (or even the *twin* of Baby 1) can manage "drowsy but awake" practically from birth, sleeps long chunks at night, naps well, and is generally just easier—and the parents have done *nothing* differently. These two babies simply have two types of wiring.

COMPARING DIFFERENT TEMPERAMENT TERMS

There are a lot of different terms used in parenting texts to refer to various constellations of temperament. They may seem like separate, standalone types, but almost all of them are rooted in the basic categories defined by original temperament researchers Alexander Thomas and Stella Chess:[8]

- *Activity level* (How physically active are they?)
- *Intensity* (How *strong* are their reactions?)
- *Rhythmicity* (How predictable are their habits, day to day?)
- *Attention span and persistence* (How focused are they on an activity? How long will they keep at it?)
- *Distractibility* (How easily can you lure them away from something they are doing or wanting?)
- *Adaptability* (How do they handle transitions or changes in routines?)
- *Approach or withdrawal* (Are they cautious? Or do they go toward new experiences?)

- *Threshold of responsiveness / reactivity* (How much input does it take to produce a response?)
- *Quality of mood* (Are they generally sunny? Or cranky / irritable?)

Their research resulted in three subgroups of temperament: easy, slow to warm up, and difficult. Most infants (75 to 80 percent), they said, were "easy," meaning they were easily soothed, and they slept and ate without a lot of fuss. "Slow to warm up" babies (about 10 percent) were cautious around strangers, new foods, and new places. They tended to hang back and observe before jumping in. The "difficult" babies (also about 10 percent) fussed and cried frequently, were harder to soothe, had trouble sleeping . . . you get the picture. The term *difficult* is still often used in research to describe these children, though *irritable*, *unsettled*, and *dysregulated* are also common.

We're not fans of these negatively skewed labels. Yes, children who cry a lot or are hard to soothe can be really, really challenging, but labeling a child "difficult" puts everyone's focus on those negative traits. In fact, there's a frustratingly large body of research on the negative repercussions of a "difficult" temperament. But what about the *good stuff* that may be right underneath or alongside the harder parts? Aren't there other ways to think about temperament and other labels we can use that might not be so black and white?

Yes. There absolutely are.

There *are* upsides to traits that can be challenging. Researchers and others just haven't spent a ton of time looking for them—and you can't find what you aren't looking for.

When we look for and identify the powerful strengths in our livewires that are mixed in with the challenges, it changes our perspective. Instead of frustration over another baffling, out-of-the-blue tantrum at Costco, you will know ahead of time that big-box stores with the crowds and lights and echoing sound are too much for your livewire. You'll know that the episode didn't come out of nowhere. They melted down, not because they're "difficult" but because their finely tuned sensory system had become overwhelmed. This shift in perception and understanding makes a huge

difference. In both scenarios, you're still trying to manage a screaming toddler in Costco, but how you *interpret* and then respond to their behavior
will be totally different. You'll make different choices. You'll plan ahead.
Maybe next time you *won't* go to the grocery store *and* Costco before naptime. You'll say different things to yourself (and them) about it.

While researchers continue to use the term *difficult* to describe these
intense kiddos, experts and authors have tried to craft some terms that also
highlight the positives. While they may sound like totally separate types,
they are really describing different clusters of traits that have a lot of overlap.
Highly sensitive children are described by author and researcher Elaine Aron
as cautious, introspective, empathic, and deeply feeling.[9] Though quieter
than their meltdown-y counterparts, these children can also be intense and
easily overwhelmed—their intensity just turns inward instead of exploding outward. William and Martha Sears refer to *high needs* babies who,
because of their more sensitive nature, need a lot of holding and carrying
and soothing.[10] Mary Sheedy Kurcinka coined the term *spirited* to describe
children who were "more" of some (or all) of the Thomas and Chess traits.[11]
Linda Budd's term *active-alert* refers to children who can be bright, intense,
and reactive.[12] All of these are great, very useful adjectives to describe the
children we're talking about in this book. We're going to use *livewire* as an
umbrella that includes all these terms because we're talking about the same
general group of kiddos—those who would not be classified as "easy."

WHAT LIVEWIRE TRAITS HAS YOUR CHILD BROUGHT TO THE PARTY?

It's important to understand what behaviors or traits are due to a livewire's
inborn nature. It's also important to know that not every livewire has the
same big traits or is off the chart in every domain. One livewire may not be
outwardly intense but they're extremely sensitive and easily overwhelmed.
Another livewire might be *very* intense and persistent but not highly active.

The following are representations of two different children and their
temperament traits. The livewire on the bottom is likely more *outwardly*

intense (note the higher scores on intensity and persistence). The livewire on the top looks like they are more emotionally sensitive (with higher scores on perceptiveness and emotional sensitivity) but not as outwardly reactive. Both children are livewires.

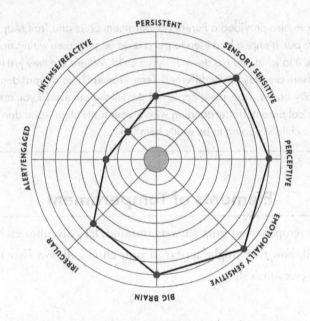

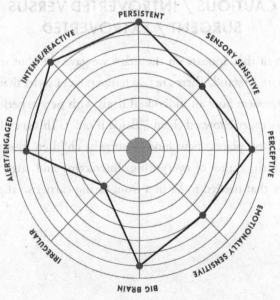

WORKBOOK TO DO

Time to fill out the Livewire Temperament Quiz and Temperament Trait Map for your livewire. Remember, they are not going to score highly on every single trait.

We've also provided a Parent Temperament Quiz and Trait Map for you to fill out. It's not a bad idea to get a read on your own wiring and then compare it to what you put down for your child. Where are they just like you? Where are they really different? Temperament is, to a great degree, genetically based. Tree, meet apple. (Note: Fill this out even if you are not a biological parent. Understanding where your traits align—and don't— with your child's is going to be really helpful.)

Elements of Temperament

With your temperament quiz answers in mind, let's dive into each trait in more detail: how they might appear in your child and how they might be impacting everyone's sleep.

CAUTIOUS / INTROVERTED VERSUS SURGENT / EXTROVERTED

This isn't a trait that appears on the maps we gave you, but it's one that's important to understand. There are two temperament styles that researchers refer to as *approach*: how an individual deals with new experiences. Some children move eagerly toward them ("Bring it on!"). This is called *surgency*. New people, new places, new foods—surgent children love them. They want to be in the center of everything, interacting and engaging. (These are the babies that needed to be in a front-facing carrier so they could see everything.) Their feelings tend to be big and loud. As these little ones get older, we would start calling them extroverts. With these big, bold little ones, their reactions are mostly directed *outward*.

Other livewires are just as intense and alert, but they move through the world differently. They are cautious and tend to wait and observe for a while before diving in. Thomas and Chess called these children "slow to warm up" because they often need time to acclimate to a new situation. Rather than rushing into the middle of the group, these livewires hang back and wait. Meltdowns can still be outwardly directed, but their intensity is often related to a depth of feeling and thinking that's more internal. Later, they are likely to be called introverts.

It's important to note that approach (or introversion / extroversion) is a continuum. If your livewire is a little of each, or changes depending on the context, that's perfectly normal. It's more important to understand that not all livewires are extroverted balls of fire. Though they still have many of the same qualities as their eager counterparts, the more cautious livewires experience things in a more internal way.

Cautious / Observant	Surgent / Outgoing
Takes time to adjust to a new environment / person	Jumps right in
Prefers to or is happy to play solo	Absolutely needs someone to interact with
Thinks a lot, doesn't talk as much	Thinks a lot, talks a lot
Socially cautious	Socially bold

INTENSITY / REACTIVITY

A livewire who is intense / reactive . . .

- Tends to experience things (happy or sad) in a big way / feels things deeeeply.
- Is easily and quickly triggered and intense crying happens fast.
- Is very easily frustrated.
- Has a fair number of crying episodes / meltdowns.
- Can be difficult to soothe or distract once upset.

Things you might have said to describe them:

"They go from zero to sixty. They're instantly in freak-out mode if I don't get to them fast."

"Everything is a big deal."

"Oh, you know what he's feeling. He really lets you know."

"Her feelings run really deep. Little things really throw her off, and it's hard for her to get back on track."

Intensity refers to the *strength* of your livewire's emotional reactions. How much power is behind their outrage, sadness, frustration, joy, or excitement? *"When they're happy, they're really happy. When they're upset . . . well, buckle up."*

Reactivity, on the other hand, refers to the *speed* of that reaction. How quickly do they get to "very upset"? *"If I don't get to them fast, they're hysterical, and it takes forever to calm them down."*

It's important to remember that we're talking about the depth, size, and speed of feeling, not to how that feeling is expressed. Quieter, more cautious livewires are as intense as those who have a more outward explosion of feeling—they just don't show it in the same way. They can still get overwhelmed by emotion (theirs or others'). For all livewires, big feelings easily zap their little regulatory systems, and meltdowns (outward) or withdrawal (inward) can happen quickly, even over positive events.

Think about emotion as an electrical current and livewires as having only a certain amount of capacity in their wiring. In real life, when you have too much current flowing through an electrical system that doesn't have enough capacity, you blow a fuse. This is what happens with livewires.

Parents often worry because, from the outside, it seems like their child just can't self-soothe . . . at all . . . ever.

It's not that livewires can't self-soothe.
They just experience larger quantities of
feelings much quicker than they can manage
with the nervous system they have.

Imagine that I handed you a twenty-pound bag of something. Chances are, you'd be able to capably hold it for a while. But if I handed you a hundred-pound bag, unless you've trained for it, you would drop it almost immediately. It's not that you don't *want* to hold the bag or that you're too lazy to hold it. You are literally not *able* because it's too heavy for the muscles you have. You are going to need help holding that bag for any length of time. Livewires' feelings and reactions are just too big for their system, and that means they need more help handling them. The good news? These big feelings eventually are a great, great strength. Livewires feel so many things so deeply and profoundly. They will likely grow to be deeply passionate, empathetic people. (I know you wonder if you will *survive* until then . . . but you will. I promise.)

How it impacts you. Let's just be real and admit that livewires' tendency to really lose it for what can feel like totally random, unknown reasons puts parents at a huge disadvantage. It can feel like you never get ahead of the freak-outs, and your days are about putting out an endless parade of emotional fires. What's worse, it can seem to others like you're overreacting. Many parents have experienced well-meaning family and friends who say, "If you keep rushing in when he cries, he'll never learn to self-soothe." Parents are made to feel guilty for helping their kiddo hold that heavy bag.

Sometimes we *do* rush in quickly—partly because we know what will happen if we don't get there fast (hell to pay), but also because enduring lots of crying does a number on anyone's nervous system. It's common for parents to want to do anything (really, *anything*) that will push pause on the screaming so there's just a little peace. This is *all of us* with livewires at some point. If this is you, you are in good company.

How it impacts sleep. Intensity / reactivity (especially the outward-facing kind) is the temperament trait that may be the *primary* driver of sleep problems for you. Livewires don't ease in and out of sleep, but spring awake and then let you *know* they're awake. It also means that *any* attempt to delay responding to "give them a chance to self-soothe" are met with explosions of crying. Who wants that in the middle of the night? We also know that once they get going, it takes even longer to get them back to calm. In calculating the cost-benefit ratios of different options, getting to them fast and doing whatever it takes to get them back to sleep is, of course, the clear winner.

Intensity / reactivity is also often the reason why sleep training didn't work or why you didn't even attempt it. Reactions to being overtired are big. Reactions to slight discomfort are big. Reactions to anything not being just right are big. If you're already worn out from current levels of intensity, it feels like a big lift to take on the drama tsunami that might happen if you tried to sleep train.

I never did sleep train because back then, it was cry it out or nothing, and I just knew what kind of fight we would be in for. Truthfully, I didn't have a lot of fight left. I just didn't have the bandwidth to face what I knew would be a battle at night. Plus, I'm a sensitive livewire, too, and I knew I couldn't hang in there with listening to her cry.

We're not going to be able to avoid intensity in this process (sorry), but we are going to do what we can to minimize it and make sure you have a clear map for navigating it.

ALERTNESS / SOCIABILITY / ENGAGEMENT

A livewire who is alert / engaged:

- Fights sleep / never seems sleepy.
- Seems like all their switches are turned on.
- Craves interaction (often at the expense of sleep).
- Rarely plays alone / independently.
- Wants a lot of contact. It may be hard or impossible to put them down.

Things you might have said to describe them:

"It's like they are just so worried they will miss out if they go to sleep."

"They're not cranky at all. They just never, ever seem sleepy and can just keep going."

"All these toys we bought . . . they only want to be on me and to see what I'm doing."

"The minute they wake up, their eyes pop open and it's like, 'game on.'"

"They're just taking it all in."

"My baby never just plays on their own . . . ever. They want me constantly."

From an early age, livewires seem to have a brain that is just "on." *Alert* babies want to be looking and seeing and experiencing—and they don't want to miss a thing. Parents of even tiny ones will say that it's impossible to get them to sleep because it's like they're worried they'll miss something. Nearly every livewire parent I've talked to will say, "It's like they have FOMO [fear of missing out]." It's so common that it's practically become a secret password to the livewire club.

I took my livewire to Disneyland when she was thirteen months old. We got a hotel room so we could go back and let her nap during the day. That never happened. She shut down the park, and at nearly 1 AM we had to give her a quiet bath just to get her excited brain to slow down. She wasn't cranky. She definitely didn't *act* overtired. She honestly could have kept going without a problem.

Sociability / engagement refers to a livewire's intense desire for interaction with interesting people or experiences. They absolutely prefer *you* to that silly play mat or other toys. Very verbal, extroverted, social livewires are going to ask questions, tell stories, share observations, make up songs. While having a child who just wants *you* can be exhausting, there are huge benefits to this level of interaction. First, they are taking in more information about actual humans. They are hearing language and getting so much exposure to interpersonal communication. Being with you (and on you) is a rich experience. By preferring interaction with you over solitary play, they also get the immense benefit of your attention and presence. They get more from you because they ask for it (require it? demand it?).

How it impacts you. There are few breaks for parents of livewires. Not only is your livewire awake for more hours in the day, but they also want to be active with *you* for those hours. Even for baby livewires who aren't yet talking, the desire to be with you instead of just chilling in a bouncy seat is strong. "Velcro babies" are attached to you at the hip and want to be wherever you are. When they're a little older and that verbal ability gets cranking, there's a fairly constant need to read books, play pretend, answer questions. It's a lot. You may find it difficult to even run to the bathroom for a moment without your livewire talking to you through the door.

How it impacts sleep. This is the trait that completely overrides any message from a livewire's little body that they need some sleep. To them, sleep is a waste of time. It's as if they see it as a sign of weakness. Naps are almost always short because the moment they move from deep sleep to light sleep, these little ones pop awake and are ready to get back to the business of learning and doing. They never seem droopy or ready for sleep. This makes them hard to read: Do they *actually* need less sleep, or do they just *act* like they do? Work on sleep is going to involve hands-on help to coax them into a pattern that will help them disengage from the exciting world to get the sleep that their busy brain needs. And while we may not be able to change their desire for you during the day, we can potentially get nighttime to be a moment when you're off the interaction clock.

PERSISTENCE

A livewire who is persistent:
- Will really dig in their heels if there's something they want.
- Can absolutely outlast you.
- Never gives up . . . ever, ever.

Things you might have said to describe them:

"Even from an early age, they knew what they wanted, and they let us know."

"There's little point in fighting. They will outlast you."

"They know what they want when they want it, and they're willing to hold out until they get it."

Persistence refers to the ability to work toward a goal, no matter what the obstacles are. And when we think about it, we *want* our children to be persistent. It's an amazing quality. But, oh boy, this is a *hard one* for parents. Livewires know what they want, and they are generally not willing to let it go. They are able to keep a goal in mind (which is good) and dig in their heels to get it (also good—inconvenient, but good).

Persistence is one of those traits whose bright side comes much farther down the road—think "teenager"—when you want them persevering and standing up for themselves. When they're young, it just feels like a fight . . . about everything . . . all the time. We are going to talk a lot more about the intensity / persistence double whammy because it plays a *huge* role in sleep and trying to get more. Trust me, there are ways to push through without breaking anyone.

How it impacts you. Livewires have a huge will, and they are prepared to outlast you. Parents can get ground down from all the conflict. When you simply can't fight for the eighteenth time in a day, what are you going to do? To others, you may appear to be "caving," but *you* know how much energy it takes to suffer through the pushback and struggle for even the simplest requests. Livewires are so strong in their desires and convictions that they wear . . . you . . . down.

How it impacts sleep. This is another trait that may have been a deal-breaker for sleep training in the past. You may absolutely know that your child can and will outlast you. I knew that sleep training for me was a nonstarter because, even if I had been willing or able to let my livewire cry before sleep, I knew it would be hours, and even then, she would never relent. For many, this isn't an abstract worry. They have tried sleep training and found out that this is completely true. It's not *just* the intensity that you're facing but the duration of that intensity and the distinct possibility that, after all of that struggle, the outcome still may not be sleep. It makes sense if, up until now, you have said no thank you to sleep training.

If you have struggled and caved and pleaded in the face of all the protest and digging in of heels, you are not alone. We've all done it . . . a lot. The problem is that, at some point, there's a feeling of powerlessness that can creep in when we start relenting because we can't face another fight. You may start to suspect that you are *incapable* of outlasting your incredibly stubborn little child. Don't be hard on yourself if this is you. We are all in this same boat to some extent.

The good news is that the work we will do on sleep will help you in more ways than you think. We are going to set a few goals and consistently push through. We'll push through sensitively, but we are going to push through. You are going to need to access your own inner reserves of persistence, but hopefully, the coming chapters will give you some confidence, some backup, and a plan. We're not trying to break your livewire's determination. No. We want them to keep *that*. However, there will be times both now and in the long-term where your will needs to be bigger than theirs. It's good for everyone to practice this. Trust me.

PERCEPTIVENESS

A livewire who is perceptive:

- Notices the slightest unusual smell, sound, movement, color, etc.
- Notices subtleties (something that's been moved, a change in a person's appearance, etc.).
- Notices any change in routines or discrepancies in limits (*"You said yes last night"*).
- Is able to compare and contrast and test out theories (*"I know you said no last night, but this is a different night"*).

Things you might have said to describe them:
"They absolutely don't miss a thing."
"Everything has to be just so or they get completely thrown off."

A perceptive child just notices . . . well, everything. They can detect subtle changes or patterns. They may recognize a symbol that they've seen, discrepancies or similarities between events or images, or patterns that you may never have detected. They will notice things that totally surprise you. My livewire, at a really young age, noticed a musical theme that occurred in two different songs in different keys in a soundtrack we were listening to. I had to go back and listen several times before I caught it. This ability to detect patterns and notice subtleties is smart stuff. Perceptiveness is a huge gift. It will keep you on your toes, parenting-wise, but wow, is it worth it.

Your livewire's gift for patterns, however, can also mean that they have a much tougher time with inconsistency or uncertainty. Too much variation or change or unpredictability throws them off much more, especially at bedtime. As a result, they appear to gravitate toward and respond well to predictability and consistency. (This knowledge will come in very handy later when we work on sleep routines.)

How it impacts sleep. When I talk to tired parents of livewires, I get the sense that they hope that maybe their livewire's sleep problems will just naturally go away or that there's some secret strategy they can use that their livewire won't even notice. When we're tired and feeling a little hopeless, we all wish there were an easier path. Unfortunately, your child's perceptiveness means that there's *nothing* that you can just sneak by them. No matter how tiny the shift, they will notice:

"We moved her favorite bear last night, and it was like the world was ending." For most livewires, a change is a change—little, big, subtle, obvious . . . doesn't matter. They see the change, they notice it, they do not like it, and because they are vocal livewires, chances are they will forcefully let you know. Or maybe you wobbled on one of your limits and allowed something "just for tonight." There's no "just for tonight" with livewires. *If it was okay last night, what's wrong with tonight or forever?* Or you worked and worked to get them to sleep without a feed and you've been at it for an hour. You decide that it's just not working and offer a bottle or a feed with the intention of trying again tomorrow. Your perceptive livewire has now clocked that a feed is an option, and their steel-trap brain will remember it (and hold you to it the next time).

How it impacts you. Having an uber perceptive little one means making sure that you are clearer and more consistent than you've ever been in your life. You may also have to be a little more rigid and predictable with routines and rules because if you're not, they will notice that tiny bit of wiggle room and you'll be stuck. Perceptiveness is just another trait to add to the list of "great stuff that makes my job a little harder."

SENSORY PROCESSING SENSITIVITY

We're going to go into a little more detail about sensory processing than some of the other temperament traits because sensory processing is at the very heart of temperament, self-soothing, and sleep. At the same time, sensory traits can be tricky to identify if you don't know to look for them. They don't always show up as "These tags are itchy," but they instead may look like hyperactivity at bedtime or that meltdown in Costco. The magic of identifying sensory processing sensitivities is that you can use this information to your advantage for sleep. At a minimum, you will be able to use sensory-based strategies that will help your livewire downshift before bedtime and avoid those that make them want to party. (And, as a bonus, you may find out that *you're* more sensory sensitive than you realize.)

Sensory processing refers to the way that the brain and nervous systems register, synthesize, and respond to sensory input from the external and internal world. Most individuals take in a level of input that their brains find easy to organize and respond to. They receive sensory information within a manageable bandwidth. Even when the input is intense (loud noises or a crowded bus), they are able to return to an even baseline within a reasonable (or even brief) amount of time.

Individuals who are sensory sensitive, on the other hand, have a system that registers and responds to input in a way that makes staying on an even keel more challenging. They experience some sensory input much more strongly. Their threshold for detecting and experiencing sensory information is quite low, and it may not take a lot for them to feel overwhelmed. Children who cover their ears when someone is chewing or hate their hair being washed or melt down in loud, busy places are *overresponsive* to sensory inputs. This kind of response is known as *sensory avoidance* or *sensory defensiveness* because these individuals may work to avoid or reduce certain levels of input to stay in balance.

Other individuals have a threshold for registering sensory information that's too high. They are *underresponsive* to some types of input and need it to be much bigger to register it. These are the children who need to be bounced on a yoga ball for sleep or crash into you with their whole body or talk / walk more loudly. These behaviors are called *sensory seeking*.

In both sensory avoiding and sensory seeking, the individual's system is working to regulate the type and amount input to maintain balance.

It's important to note that individuals are not globally over- or underresponsive to *all* types of sensory input. Some sensory modalities may be more of a challenge than others. For example, a child may be incredibly sensitive to light touch but not bothered at all by loud noises. Individuals can also be a mix of these styles: sensory seeking in one type of input and sensory avoiding in another. Keep this in mind when you look at the lists below.

A livewire who is overresponsive (sensory avoiding):

- Is distressed by certain fabrics or textures, new tastes, or textures of food.
- Is bothered by light touch (like stroking or lightly patting).
- Dislikes the bath, getting their hair washed, or diaper changes.
- Becomes upset in crowded places (malls, warehouse stores, etc.).
- Is sensitive to noises that most children are not bothered by (fans, voices, vacuum cleaners, sirens, etc.).
- Needs their room to be completely dark and/or quiet to sleep and wakes up at the slightest noise or light.

A livewire who is underresponsive (sensory seeking):

- Is extremely attached to their pacifier (can't calm down without it).
- Needs excessive movement for sleep (swinging, bouncing, etc.).
- Likes to be swaddled tightly or have full-body contact to fall asleep; if older, they like to have heavy blankets, lots of stuffed animals, or tighter pajamas.
- Needs consistent sound or white noise to stay asleep.
- If older, likes to crash into things, push against you, or jump around at bedtime.
- Chews on their sleeves, hair, or toy and likes crunchy or sour foods.

Sensory processing involves eight senses (yes, eight): the five that we're super familiar with—sight, sound, taste, smell, and touch—plus three more that you may not know as much about—proprioception, vestibular input, and interoception. Lindsey Biel, coauthor of *Raising a Sensory Smart Child*, explains:

> *Proprioceptive input* from the joints, muscles, and connective tissues of our bodies gives us body awareness so we can develop an internal map of where all of our body parts are in space. *Vestibular input* from sensory receptors in the inner ear tell us about how we are moving. These two senses work together like a GPS, so we know where we are and how we are moving at all times. Finally, there is *interoception* which gives us (largely unconscious) awareness of the physiological state of our bodies such as hunger, thirst, fatigue, heart rate, respiration rate, and bowel and bladder status.

According to Biel, all eight of our senses "*ideally* integrate seamlessly and automatically. However, for some, all this sensory information gets registered and integrated in a different way, so the person does not have the expected responses to sensory experiences."[13]

More-sensitive individuals take in a lot more information through their senses and then have trouble synthesizing or processing it. Too much or the wrong kind of input can overwhelm a livewire's ability to stay on a physiological even keel. Remember the analogy of holding that heavy bag? This is similar. When sensory systems are overwhelmed, the ability to stay calm breaks down.

This breakdown might *look* like a tantrum—a strategy meant to make you change your mind about something they wanted—but it's actually a *sensory meltdown*. These are much bigger than tantrums and almost feel like a storm that comes over your child. They may seem a little out of their mind with it, and it's nearly impossible to stop once it's started. Meltdowns are a sign that your child's sensory system has become overwhelmed (the circuit breaker has been tripped), and they are going to need your help to reset the system.

There are lots of factors that influence a child's ability to manage sensory input or disruptions: how well they're eating and sleeping, how many transitions and stressors are occurring at any given time, and more. For some children, little bumps in the road can really add up—another child bumped into them in line at daycare, they had to go with you to Target, they skipped their nap. Biel says, "These factors accumulate throughout the day (and night), making it seem like your child has had a meltdown seemingly out of nowhere."

How it impacts you. Sensory processing is the key to so many struggles you may be having with your livewire. You may wonder *Why is riding in the car such a nightmare? Why do they freak out when I'm trying to wash their hair? Why do I have to bounce on a ball like a maniac to get them to sleep?* Sensory processing sensitivities are not easy to figure out on your own. As Biel notes, "It is essential to work with experts who can help build a stronger system so that your child can increasingly manage the many experiences of a sensory world."[14] An assessment from a pediatric occupational therapist (OT) can help you understand your child's sensory strengths and challenges and can provide exercises, strategies, and modification solutions to help improve their ability to regulate and tolerate different input.

How it impacts sleep. How *doesn't* it impact sleep? Research has shown some clear links between sensory sensitivities and challenges with sleep.[15] Being able to buffer out sounds and sensations and fall asleep is not always in a sensory-sensitive livewire's wheelhouse. Their pajamas are too loose, the room is too cold or too quiet, they didn't get enough energy out before bedtime. There are so many ways that sensory sensitivities can really do a number on the ability to fall asleep and stay asleep. We'll talk later in chapter eight about some sensory strategies that can work for bedtime and sleep.

ADAPTABILITY / FRUSTRATION TOLERANCE

A livewire who is unadaptable / has low frustration tolerance:

- Has a lot of difficulty (meltdowns) with abrupt changes (*"We have to leave now"*) and needs *lots* of warning before a transition (bedtime, leaving the playground, etc.).
- Has a lot of difficulty when a task or a goal isn't achieved.
- Is easily and strongly frustrated by an unexpected event (*"We're out of cereal"*).
- Responds well to predictability and super consistent routines with clear cues.
- May have difficulty sleeping anywhere but in their familiar spot.

Livewires can have a *very* low tolerance for unexpected changes. Disruptions or surprises can really throw them off and cause a level of uncertainty that they *do not* like. Unadaptable livewires need a ton of warning before any change that is going to happen. Some livewires also have a hair trigger for frustration. I've heard from many parents about walking on eggshells and not quite knowing what might set their little one off. Nonadaptable livewires don't seem to be able to shift gears when their expectations get upended. Something as simple as *"No, we can't read an extra book"* or *"Dad is going to do the routine instead tonight"* can be the source of an hour-long freak-out. Meltdowns happen because these livewires can't switch gears on the fly. They need time, and they need warning. Otherwise, out-of-the-blue changes blow their circuits.

To be honest, adaptability and low frustration tolerance don't have a totally perfect upside. They just seem to be a by-product of sensitive wiring. The best we can do when change or disruption is inevitable is to offer support, take their need for advance warning into account, and help them get a little better at navigating frustrating situations.

How it impacts sleep. Low frustration tolerance and nonadaptability really impact the process of changing sleep patterns, rather than impacting sleep itself. Trying to change a livewire's familiar patterns can be met with so . . . much . . . pushback. They really hate change. Like with persistence, there's really no way around this. What we can do is accept that they don't like change, prepare them for the new pattern, and support them through the hard moments as we push through to the other side. If we can hang in there, livewires do seem to settle in once a new pattern feels familiar and stable.

How it impacts you. This is another hard trait for parents. With easygoing children, parents can say, "How about we do this now instead?" The child may grumble, but they go along. With livewires, it's like you've asked them to move a mountain. Every request or unexpected change is usually a massive deal. It can be exhausting and wears on the old patience reserves.

If your child needs time to shift gears or wrap their head around an unexpected turn of events, you knowing this will inform both how you approach those events and how you interpret your livewire's response. When you've promised a slushie after you get through Target and they're out of blue raspberry and there's a half-hour meltdown because that's the flavor that they planned for (true story) . . . well, at least you know why.

EMOTIONAL SENSITIVITY

A livewire who is emotionally sensitive:
- Notices and reacts to the distress or feelings of others.
- Responds strongly to discipline or correction.
- Feels things deeply.
- Notices social dynamics (exclusion, bullying, conflict, etc.).
- Is precociously intuitive or insightful.

Livewires are almost always very deeply feeling little beings. Their perceptive nature makes them highly attuned to others' feelings. Even as infants, they can appear to pick up on their parents' moods. When they're a little older, they can be very aware of social dynamics. In school, these are the children who befriend peers who are left out. They are outraged by bullying or mean behavior. When that behavior is directed toward them, they can be deeply wounded.

How it impacts sleep. A livewire's exquisite sensitivities make them brilliant and empathic and creative. When they're old enough, this depth of feeling can also make them more vulnerable to worries or sadness over events that happened that day or that they happened to hear about. These thoughts and feelings can roar to the surface at bedtime just when you're about to say good night. For older children, overthinking is a common bedtime challenge. We're going to talk about not only ways to help them put all these thoughts on hold at nighttime but also how to teach them some self-calming, self-affirming strategies that will help in the long-term.

How it impacts you. Having a little one with very deep feelings can mean that you are doing a lot more processing and reframing of everyday events—something they heard on television, for example, or something a friend said to them at the park. They may worry about issues that are beyond their years. Their emotional antennae are up *all the time*, and they will need you to buffer out as much as you can, then provide support and guidance when you can't.

ACTIVITY LEVEL

A livewire who is highly active:

- Has two speeds: asleep and go, go, go.
- Is an Energizer Bunny—never stops.
- Is early on most or all motor milestones: rolling, crawling, standing, walking.
- Has a Houdini-like ability to get out of cribs, rooms, sleep sacks, swaddles, etc.

Some livewires are not only mentally super active but also constantly on the move . . . like, *constantly*. This high activity level often goes along with some physical or athletic ability. These are the kiddos who are climbing out of their crib or up the bookshelves and dresser way before they should be able to. They figure out baby-gate latches and how to extract themselves from sleep sacks. Or they may just be running and jumping and zooming the whole time they are awake. Parents of an active livewire may worry that their child has ADHD when, in reality, they are just popping with mental and physical energy.

How it impacts sleep. The challenge of getting them to sleep may be figuring out how to get them to slow down long enough to sleep and then how to keep them in their room or bed without locking them in there.

How it impacts you. High activity levels mean you are going to be pooped from chasing after them, keeping them engaged, and keeping them safe.

IRREGULARITY / UNPREDICTABILITY

A livewire who is irregular / unpredictable:
- Has no reliable pattern of eating or sleeping.
- Does not respond in a predictable way to your sleep strategies (something works for a few days then stops).

Some children are like clockwork. You can practically set your watch by their meal and nap times. With irregular or unpredictable livewires, however, their eating, sleeping, and bathroom patterns seem to change day to day. They may also have very irregular responses to parenting strategies: what works one day absolutely does not the very next day. Parents will say, "Nothing changed! I did the exact same thing I did yesterday, and it worked like a charm. Today? Total fail."

How it impacts you. Irregularity is something that parents often don't realize is related to temperament, but it truly is. A lack of predictability can be challenging, for sure, because it makes it hard to know what to expect. Sleep strategies work for a couple of days, then don't anymore. Or your livewire magically slept through the night one day, you have no earthly idea why, and then they don't again. It's frustrating. It's super puzzling. It also can make you feel like you don't have any impact on your child's behavior. The best that we can do in these circumstances is help *you* feel like you understand your end of it—what you're responsible for. Then, whatever roundabout, out-of-left-field behavior your livewire may throw at you is what it is. At least *you* can be consistent and predictable even if they're not (right now).

How it impacts sleep. Unpredictability makes working on new sleep habits tricky. Parents with unpredictable livewires already feel like there's no rhyme or reason to why a particular day is a good sleep day or a bad one. It may be like this as we move forward, too. Improvement may not go in a straight line. We're going to talk about this in more detail later, but don't let ups and downs in the process throw you. That's how your livewire rolls. It doesn't mean that *we* can't keep going. In fact, you will need to, despite their unpredictable response.

BIG BRAIN

A supersmart livewire:

- Is intuitive or empathic.
- Has a very early interest in language or books.
- Has an early intense interest in a specific subject / activity (drawing, dinosaurs, etc.).
- Is very verbal / talks a lot / talks early.
- Is very observant (notices subtle patterns or details).
- Hits motor milestones ahead of schedule.
- Values justice / fairness / ethical behavior.
- Can appear "bossy" / knows how they want things to be / what they want to happen.
- Tends to be a perfectionist / wants everything "just so."
- Can be divergent and independent (marches to their own drummer and thinks outside the box).

Okay, hang on tight—I'm going to talk about intelligence.

Whenever I start talking about the g-word (*giftedness*), parents start getting nervous. Bear with me. If you look at what researchers have, at least theoretically, defined as early signs of a powerful brain,[16] there are startling overlaps with some of the temperament traits we see in livewires:

- Early alertness (at birth and just after)
- High activity level
- Early interest in books / language
- High degree of perceptiveness
- Emotional sensitivity

One of my graduate students and I conducted some research with parents of identified gifted school-age children where we asked what they were like as infants. A shocking number of parents mentioned the traits I just listed—but also awful sleep problems, difficulty with self-soothing, meltdowns, sensory sensitivities, etc. The overlaps were surprising and significant.[17]

Another way to talk about early indicators of intelligence is in terms of *overexcitabilities* or OEs, which is a more global kind of intelligence.[18] OEs qualitatively differ from our notion of IQ, which measures academic ability. They refer to extra aptitude or interest in a variety of areas: sensory (appreciation of music, art, language, food, etc.), imaginative, physical (athleticism, agility, dance), intellectual (intense curiosity, interest in many areas), and emotional (empathic, intuitive, ethical). The description of this kind of intelligence strongly overlaps the kinds of behaviors and traits we see even in very young livewires.

It's therefore possible that intelligence and creativity are the biggest upsides to a challenging temperament. Livewires know more and feel more than they can manage at younger ages. It just makes sense that all the drama is merely a by-product of a powerful brain in a little body.

How it impacts sleep. Sometimes, it takes time and work to get a busy brain to slow down enough to be ready for sleep. The desire to be interacting and learning and doing is so strong. Bedtime is a time when the brain can keep spinning with stories and questions and ideas. Worries from the day get bigger. Shadows in the dark room look like monsters. In chapter eight, we will talk at length about strategies that will help a livewire quiet their brain and body so that they can turn their attention toward getting some rest.

How it impacts you. Children with active brains require a lot from parents—keeping them stimulated and busy, protecting them from input that could be distressing (and start an avalanche of worry and questions), helping them navigate peer relationships, and more. Shepherding these forces of nature through childhood is epic superhero-level stuff.

PUTTING IT ALL TOGETHER

Understanding the elements of temperament gives you critical information without which you can end up swimming upstream when it comes to sleep. Knowing your child's temperament strengths and challenges means you can work *with* them instead of against them. It can also help you take their shenanigans less personally. Knowing the source of their behavior lets you think through better ways to address it.

Each of your livewire's phenomenal abilities *directly* impacts how sleep happens (or doesn't). Having a solid handle on both the upsides and challenges of their temperament will tell you a lot about how you may need to adjust your sleep strategies so that you are harnessing their abilities, rather than fighting against them. This will be at the heart of our work and the way that you will finally get some traction on improving sleep. We are going to put your child's livewire traits front and center, where they need to be.

OUR TRIP CHECKLIST

☑ You know you are on a different path.

☑ You understand your livewire's temperament strengths and challenges.

☐ You understand the link between temperament and sleep issues.

☐ Your child is ready:

    ☐ Over six months

    ☐ No upcoming disruptions

    ☐ No physiological issues that affect sleep

☐ You are ready (or as ready as you can be).

☐ You understand the Big Four sources of sleep issues.

☐ Big Strategy #1: You know how to avoid that second wind.

☐ Big Strategy #2: You have a solid, consistent bedtime routine.

☐ Big Strategy #3 and #4: You know how to change the go-to-sleep and back-to-sleep patterns and are prepared to be more consistent than you've ever been before.

☐ You know how to track progress.

☐ You know how to diagnose and fix any problems that arise.

☐ BETTER SLEEP!

CHAPTER 3

You Are Here: Why Is Sleep So Hard?

Children who are good sleepers (dandelions) appear to have a hardwired ability to power down when they're tired and ignore any outside noise or sensations. This is true for adults as well as children. Think about the last time you were on an overnight flight. You could immediately tell the good sleepers (sitting up, arms folded, dead to the world) from the non-sleepers (eye mask, headphones, blanket, pillow, still not asleep). Why would babies or children be any different?

Livewires have more trouble with just about every aspect of sleep because of how they are wired. Sleep is harder to get and harder to maintain. For non-livewires, the road to sleep may not be a complete cakewalk, but it's straighter, flatter, and shorter than the one you're on. I'm not going to lie: Your path is harder, steeper, and rockier and requires more skill, preparation, and stamina. You are going to need different tools, a better map, and a much bigger survival kit. Here's the cool part: We're going to help you get them, and it's going to change everything. Understanding how temperament can affect the process of sleep is the first step to figuring out what's been getting in the way. It's a game-changer.

HOW A LIVEWIRE TEMPERAMENT
MAKES SLEEP AN UPHILL CLIMB

Falling asleep (even when you're *really* tired) involves several steps that you may not be fully conscious of. If you've ever had insomnia, you *know* how difficult falling asleep can be. The ability to go to sleep has a lot to do with tuning in to internal signals and tuning out external ones. So, what does it take to fall asleep, and why do livewires have so much trouble with it?

1. You have to notice that you feel tired / sleepy.

When it's time to power down for a rest, the body sends out biochemical signals to help you slow down and fall asleep. Most children detect and respond to those signals. They yawn. They rub their eyes. They look droopy. They *feel* sleepy. They get cranky.

As the parent of a livewire, you might be thinking, *What's this "yawning" thing you're talking about? I've never seen it. "Looking tired"? Never heard of it.*

Livewires do not get the memo from their brain that they need a break. It's hard to know whether this is because the signals are weaker or because livewires are just so busy that they don't pay attention to them. Some parents say that their bright, active livewire seems to need less sleep than other children. We're not convinced that's true. In our experience, livewires don't need less sleep. They just *act* like they do.

Here's what I know about livewire sleepy signals:

- If you are waiting for a sleepy signal, you may be waiting a *long* time.
- If you *do* see a yawn or an eye rub, you might already be too late. (Can you say "second wind"?)

Needless to say, we will not be waiting for sleepy signals to tell us that it's time for sleep, and at least at first, we will shoot for the age-appropriate sleep targets. More about this in chapter seven.

2. You have to be willing and able to disconnect from the waking world.

Typically, once a tired signal is sent and is detected by the brain, the body starts to downshift to sleep by taking sensory and thought-processing systems offline for a bit and turning attention away from external input to turn toward sleep.

Well, this one is just nearly impossible for livewires. Their desire to be interacting with the world overrides their need for rest. Even when they are in the crib or bed and getting ready to sleep, these livewires can fight it with all they've got. Parents have told me that their newborn will be on the brink of sleep, eyes half-closed, only to force their eyes back open to keep looking around. Or their toddler who just can't stop thinking about the new story idea they have and *has to* tell them about it *right now*. Amazing, yes? They are so invested in their waking experiences that they just don't want to give them up, even when they're really pooped.

Parents will say, "It's like they just don't want to waste time with sleep. They want to be doing." How incredible! Think of how much this livewire is taking in and how much they're learning. But this is exactly why the deck is stacked differently for parents of livewires. Sleep is a much bigger mountain to climb, and you have to drag your child up it with you.

3. You have to be able to ignore or tune out external stimuli.

All that good sleepers need for sleep are soft jammies, a firm mattress, and a somewhat darkened room because their sleep drive has them halfway to Sleepytown by the time they get into bed. Noise, temperature, pacifier / no pacifier . . . it doesn't really matter. It takes just a little effort and—*poof*! They're asleep. For livewires, it can be like "The Princess and the Pea." Tiiiny sensations from the environment—light, sound, temperature, a wrinkle in the sheet—can shift their attention *away* from sleep and *back* to the world. These are babies that pop awake the second you lay them in the crib or toddlers whose eyes fly open as soon as you start to ninja your way out of the room, even though you were *sure* they were finally asleep. Even when co-sleeping, a sneeze, the sound of a sheet moving, or the motion of the bed as someone turns over can be too much. Livewires struggle big time with *every* aspect of the journey from awake to asleep. They don't detect signals that they *should* (tiredness), and they can't help but pay attention to input that they should *ignore* (light, temperature, sound). Sleep challenges exist because, for livewires, the road from awake to asleep is long, hard, and full of detours.

WHY THE USUAL CRY IT OUT APPROACHES DON'T WORK

The difficulties livewires have with the transition into sleep, as well as their sensitivity to the environment, are the big culprits in the lack of success you may have had with the usual sleep training methods. Remember, sleep books are written primarily for dandelions, who have much less trouble disconnecting and falling asleep.

Here are the major components of the standard sleep training advice you may have encountered and why they don't work for livewires.

Strike #1: Put your baby down "drowsy but awake."

Experts advise parents to put their baby down in the bassinet drowsy but awake practically from birth so they can practice falling asleep without nursing or rocking. Cool, cool. For livewires, this advice is a complete non-starter. So many parents have told me about their struggles with trying to put their baby down *not* fully asleep: *"The books never say what to do when the baby goes ballistic. There's no 'falling asleep' happening."* The ability to go from drowsy to asleep on a separate, firm surface is a skill that doesn't fully kick in for most babies (even dandelions) until about six months, and for livewires, it might be even later. Because of sensory processing sensitivities, alertness, and intensity, going to sleep without movement or other help can be very, very difficult, if not impossible.

Strike #2: Delay responding to crying, and children will learn to self-soothe.

While children's ability to manage distress grows as they do, livewires can still struggle with emotional regulation despite their increasing developmental skills. Livewires have so much more emotional and sensory current running through their system that there's simply more for them to try to manage. The skills they have are no match for the big and fast tidal wave of reaction that they can experience. Parents often tell me, "If I don't get to her immediately, we're in for an hour of crying." They also know that waiting to see if their emotional powerhouse will calm back down on their own is a dead end. Livewires don't relent and stop crying. They get *more* upset because their level of emotion has surpassed what they can handle. They know they need help, and they know they need it from you.

Some pediatricians and experts like to say that offering help just overstimulates children or reinforces the crying and prevents them from developing self-soothing skills. While it makes sense not to *over*respond (it's important for children to practice experiencing some tolerable frustration), withholding help when a child really needs it so that they'll "learn" doesn't make sense—and with livewires it never really works. (There's also no evidence that helping a child calm down is overstimulating or gets in the way of learning self-regulation skills.)

Strike #3: It will only take a few days of crying.

This is potentially the biggest stumbling block for parents of livewires who have tried cry it out–based sleep training methods. For livewires, it's often *not* only a few days but weeks . . . and it's often not only crying but hysterics—screaming, vomiting, losing their voice. Some books say that that doesn't matter, you just keep going. But . . . seriously? There is a vast difference between fifteen to twenty minutes of crying before the child goes to sleep and an hour or more of full-on disorganized, head-spinning turmoil every night for over a week or more. Books and the research they cite are simply not talking about the level or duration of crying that livewires and their parents can experience. It should be noted, too, that even in research, cry it out often took weeks to work.[19] This idea that it works in just a couple of days is only true for a small number of parents.

EXCLUSIVELY "FOLLOWING CUES" AND CO-SLEEPING MAY NOT WORK, EITHER

Many parents have never even attempted cry it out approaches because either they don't agree with it or they know ahead of time it would be a total bust. The alternative for some is to follow their child's cues and respond as needed. I hate to tell you this, but that strategy *also* may not work for you quite the way the books say it should. Don't get me wrong—I'm a *huge* proponent of being responsive to needs and to distress. I went all in on the "just follow cues" route with both of my livewires and really hoped that if I just kept following them, things would even out and they would gradually learn to sleep better. For me, and for many of the parents I've worked with, this didn't happen. Even co-sleeping wasn't the answer. For me, it was preferable to the alternative, but most days, it was rock meet hard place.

The good news is that your choices aren't only cry it out or gut it out. We're offering an alternative method to shifting your child's sleep patterns, one that adopts a gradual approach that doesn't overwhelm your livewire's abilities by causing a ton of distress but nevertheless encourages them to stretch a little and learn new skills. We promise it can be done.

Here's where we're going to diverge from the other sleep advice:

- We're going to fully understand how *your* livewire's temperament affects both sleep and how they respond to change.
- We're going to rule out anything that could stand in the way of success (especially if it's something that should be assessed before you start).
- We're going to make sure that *you* feel ready and confident.
- We're going to identify and tackle the easiest parts first (yes, there are some easy steps that really make a difference).

- We're going to do everything we can to help you set up the day and bedtime so that your livewire is as ready as they can be for sleep.

Then, we'll look at what you can do to facilitate better sleep skills. It may feel like we're covering a lot of ground before we get to working on sleep, but there's a lot of planning and prep that goes into a road trip before you head out. You figure out where you need to go and what routes are best to take you there. The car has to be serviced and full of gas. Essentials have to be packed (map, snacks, toolbox, flares). It can take some time before you finally hit the road—but just like with a road trip, you will be glad you planned ahead. I mean, this road is bumpy enough. Let's make sure you are really set up for success.

OUR TRIP CHECKLIST

- ☑ You know you are on a different path.
- ☑ You understand your livewire's temperament strengths and challenges.
- ☑ You understand the link between temperament and sleep issues.
- ☐ Your child is ready:
  - ☐ Over six months
  - ☐ No upcoming disruptions
  - ☐ No physiological issues that affect sleep
- ☐ You are ready (or as ready as you can be).
- ☐ You understand the Big Four sources of sleep issues.
- ☐ Big Strategy #1: You know how to avoid that second wind.
- ☐ Big Strategy #2: You have a solid, consistent bedtime routine.
- ☐ Big Strategy #3 and #4: You know how to change the go-to-sleep and back-to-sleep patterns and are prepared to be more consistent than you've ever been before.
- ☐ You know how to track progress.
- ☐ You know how to diagnose and fix any problems that arise.
- ☐ BETTER SLEEP!

Is Everybody Ready?

CHAPTER 4

Is Your Livewire Ready?

Believe it or not, not every child is ready for working on sleep. We want to make sure that you're not starting this journey with a great big roadblock in the way that's going to make things even harder than they need to be. The more obstacles we can move out of the way, the easier the road will be. Here are some important questions to answer before you start.

PLEASE HOLD: IS YOUR CHILD YOUNGER THAN SIX MONTHS?

» *If the answer is no, you can skip to page 73.*

There are tons of experts who will tell you that if you start off right from birth with putting them in the crib "drowsy but awake," you will get good habits going and prevent problems from happening. Mmm . . . maybe? If you have a little one who is wired for sleep right out of the gate, great sleep at early ages can happen—but not because a parent put them down drowsy but awake. If this method worked for someone you know, I guarantee they have an easygoing child who is wired to navigate the transition to sleep without much trouble. You, the other hand, can try "drowsy but awake" all day long with your livewire, and it won't necessarily translate to better sleep.[20]

There's also *no research* on the need for or benefit of starting early. None. Nada. And no one has looked at whether it's any harder or less effective to wait until the baby is older. Research on preventing sleep problems in very young babies often found that improvements were very small[21]—and also wore off in just a few months.[22] The bottom line is that working on sleep skills at this age likely only helps babies who are already competent sleepers. For *most* infants (and with livewires, for sure), actual sleep training at early ages has no perceptible benefit—and honestly, just ratchets up the pressure on parents.

Given all of that, hang on to your hat:

We're going to suggest that—if at all possible— you wait to actively intervene in your child's sleep until closer to six months.

Why? If you can hold off on working on sleep behaviors until your baby is a little older, you may find that it's actually *easier*, and you'll have more traction. After six months, sleep has moved into a more organized structure, the chaos of the four-month sleep regression has settled down, and babies have more tools in their self-regulation toolbox. Parents often instinctively know this, but because of the warnings they get from experts, they feel wrong (or weak) for feeling like they should wait. When I tell the parents of younger livewires that they can put off worrying about sleep skills for now and that everything they're doing is developmentally appropriate (and easier on everyone), I can almost see the weight of anxiety lifting off their shoulders. Yes, it is okay to wait, and it's okay to do what works for now.

You cannot create "bad habits" that can't be shifted later.

Self-soothing takes time to develop.

According to most child-rearing advice, self-soothing (especially when it comes to sleep) is something that a child only learns if you *don't* respond to distress. This is such a funny notion when you think about it. We don't talk about *any* other childhood skill in this way. No one says, "Don't carry your baby. If you carry them, they will become dependent on it and they will never learn to walk." We know that a very young baby cannot walk and there's no point in withholding appropriate help. I may be exaggerating a little . . . but not a lot. I've had lots of parents who don't want to feed or hold their tiny new baby to sleep because they're afraid they will start dependencies that will block the development of self-soothing. Sleep is the *one* arena where experts claim that learning will only happen if we don't help.

Self-soothing means that an individual is *doing* something to make themselves feel better. Let's think about what you do to calm down when you are really upset. You may call a friend, go on a run or to the gym, go to a movie, punch a pillow, meditate, write in a journal, etc. As an adult, you have a *ton* of options—all of which require that you are able to think about the issue, problem-solve, and then act on your choices.

Babies have way fewer options. What can they actually *do*? Older babies and toddlers can find their pacifier or lovey, suck their fingers or thumb, stroke their own hair, or shift their gaze to something that will distract them. Younger infants can't rely on motor skills to competently get their hand to their mouth. They can't even shift their attention away from the distress. And for livewires, who feel everything more strongly, their distress is going to quickly become more than they can handle. Because their little regulation toolbox is virtually empty, the amount of distress they can capably handle on their own is really, really small. They need help calming down.

Rather than learning self-soothing in the *absence* of help, developmental scientists and experts in the field of affective neuroscience (the biology of emotional development) suggest that soothing is learned *in relationship* with loving caregivers across the first several years of childhood.[23] They call this co-regulation.[24] In the early months, your consistent presence and help with soothing shows your child what it *feels like* to go from distressed to calm or sleepy to asleep or alert to drowsy.[25] Once they have that felt experience, their nervous system has a template for regulation that they can access later as their skills develop. Like everything else in childhood, we help our children until they can do it more independently.

What can you do before six months? The short answer is: whatever works. Everything we typically do to make sleep easier (holding, rocking, feeding) is all on the table. (For more detailed, developmentally based information on sleep in the first few months, check out Kim's book *The Sleep Lady's Gentle Newborn Sleep Guide*.)

What if sleep is really bad before six months?

There's "normal" waking for young infants (say, two to three times a night), and then there's "waking every hour." Even for a livewire, that's a lot. When a baby's behavior far exceeds even the upper end of normal, it's time to ask why. When babies are persistently fussy (like *all* the time), there generally is a reason. If your baby seems uncomfortable or just not happy even when you are holding or lying with them, a bigger issue may be at hand.

Some pediatricians are inclined to believe that sleep training is the answer to most of parents' concerns about fussy or sleepless babies, or they hesitate to treat a baby in case parents are merely overreacting. If you *know* there is something wrong, don't be afraid to push for a more careful assessment or switch providers. I've seen too many parents with babies who were really suffering be told that the child would grow out of it or that it's normal or that their baby was "just fussy." *Just fussy?* That's like being told, "It's just a compound fracture. Take some ibuprofen and ice it." If you feel in your gut that your baby is fussier than they should be or you *know* something is wrong, it's okay to push.

Possible physiological culprits of sleep problems in babies under six months

A lot of fussiness or waking every hour or two are (almost always) signs of something physical going on. With babies this young, it's even more important to double-check feeding, digestion, and other body-centered events that prevent a baby from feeling comfortable enough to sleep.

Feeding issues. In the first six months, feeding has more influence on sleep than anything else. Structural problems, like a lip / tongue tie, or other conditions can impact food intake and result in babies being hungry more frequently or taking in air that gets trapped in their tummies. Hungry or uncomfortable babies will wake a lot. Check with a lactation consultant if you are at all concerned about how much your baby is eating and when.

Silent reflux. Silent reflux is often a primary culprit when we see serious sleep and crying problems in our practices. A large number of babies who have "colic" (inconsolable crying for hours a day) are actually suffering from reflux (with spitting up) or silent reflux (no spitting up). Silent reflux is like baby heartburn. Stomach acid bubbles up into the esophagus and can cause pain. Some possible symptoms besides persistent crying and sleep issues include:

- Persistent fussiness (just not happy, especially at night)
- Crying hard or a lot when lying flat (especially after a feed)
- Preferring to sleep on an incline (in arms, in a seat, etc.) or on their side
- Grimacing (like they have a bad taste in their mouth), throat clearing, or a gurgling sound in the throat
- "Nibble nursing" (only taking a little bit, frequently) or nursing best while drowsy
- Arching their back while nursing

Silent reflux can be a significant event for everyone. It's important to get it checked by a pediatrician and treated, if necessary. Reducing a baby's pain around eating and sleeping can bring stress down significantly. Once reflux is better managed, sleep may improve a bit all by itself.

Physical (musculoskeletal) discomfort. Believe it or not, infants can have lingering physical effects from the birth process—pinched or tight muscles and misalignment, including torticollis. Silent reflux and latch or feeding issues can also cause the body to tense, which can cause pain while lying in a bassinet or other surface. Pediatric chiropractors or craniosacral therapists specialize in these physical issues. Just like it would be for us adults, when lying on their back is painful for a baby, or a tight neck muscle prevents them from moving freely, sleep is going to be hard. Getting these symptoms addressed can sometimes be miraculous in terms of improving a baby's comfort and ability to sleep.

The magic of the six-month mark: Why it's helpful to wait

In the early months of a baby's life, sleep patterns are really variable and there are big differences among individual babies.[26] By six months, however, sleep shifts into a new level of organization. Short, frequent naps consolidate into three predictable(ish) longer naps, and bedtime becomes less variable. This means you are able to create a sleep schedule that allows for a predictable, earlier start to their nighttime sleep (that leaves a little time for you to be a grown-up individual human before you have to go to bed, too).

Babies are also able to go longer without feeds and do more of the work of going to sleep with a little less help than before. They are now able to roll to sleep on their tummy if they get uncomfortable on their back, and they are more adept at getting their fingers or hand to their mouth if they want.

By waiting until your livewire has more skills in their developmental toolbox, you have a better chance of really moving the needle on sleep. Six months is also often when parents are ready to move the crib out of their room. For livewires, this is a great time to start with a new approach to sleep: new room, new sleep strategy.

STOP, DO NOT PASS GO: RULING OUT POTENTIAL ROADBLOCKS (FOR SIX MONTHS AND UP)

There are a few important and common reasons to wait on making this sleep trek even if your livewire is older than six months. Sleep training is hard enough. We don't want you putting in a ton of effort when there's a massive boulder in the way.

Big life changes: Proceed with caution

Before you begin sleep coaching, it's important to have a clear schedule, with a month or two before any big disruptions (travel, new sibling, moving, etc.). Better sleep won't take *that* long, but big changes can cause sleep routines to wobble. Remember that livewires are good at detecting alterations in their usual routine, and they do not love change. Older livewires can see change as an opportunity to negotiate new patterns (*"The baby gets to sleep in with Mom and Dad. Now, I want to, too."*). You definitely don't want to have to start all over again after the disruption. When starting a new pattern, you really want to give it time to take root. Plan accordingly.

Note: Regressions and teething are not necessarily considered roadblocks because if you wait for a break in either of them, you'll be waiting a long time.

Checking under the hood: Ruling out physiological causes of sleep issues

Underlying physiological issues are a main cause of big, persistent problems with sleep regardless of age and, for babies and young children, lead to a lack of any success with sleep training efforts. Livewires are so sensitive to any physiological discomfort that it doesn't take much to throw them off, and trying to work on sleep when there's a physical culprit always results in a battle. Fussiness, crying, stalling, and not wanting to lie down may look like garden-variety shenanigans, but they can also be related to something physical that's causing the behavior. If this is the case, you could work on sleep until the cows come home and sleep wouldn't budge. We want to be 100 percent sure that *nothing else* explains why your little one is struggling so hard with sleep.

Ruling out possible underlying issues will also help *you* feel confident that nothing else is going on. Being uncertain about whether your livewire has an undiagnosed issue will throw a monkey wrench of doubt into the process, and you'll have a hard time feeling confident and being consistent.

> **IMPORTANT CAVEAT:** The information below is not meant to diagnose conditions. You should *always* check with your pediatrician or other medical provider for input, assessment, and diagnosis.

Low ferritin, pediatric restless legs syndrome, and periodic limb movement disorder

Ferritin is a protein in the blood that helps store the iron that's in the bloodstream. An individual can have enough iron in their blood (something that typically gets tested at your pediatrician's office), but if ferritin is low, the body is not able to store and then use that iron.

Low ferritin is a little-known cause of very difficult and intractable sleep problems. Low ferritin can cause restless sleep, prolonged time to fall asleep, or periods of wakefulness in the middle of the night. In adults, low ferritin causes restless legs syndrome (RLS)—a misleading name, as it just sounds like you want to move your legs. You *do*, but the "restless" part is because the uncomfortable (sometimes painful) sensations involved in RLS are only relieved by movement. I recently encountered a dad who didn't realize he had RLS until we started discussing his livewire. The dad said that every night at bedtime, he felt like he wanted to "cut his own legs off" because of the discomfort. So, it's a little more intense than just restlessness. Older children can report that their legs feel painful or jumpy. I had one eight-year-old who said he just felt "nervous."

Identifying low ferritin in infants and toddlers is more difficult simply because their difficulty with sleep can look like a variety of things. There is actually a big overlap between RLS and what we usually call growing pains—so much so that doctors suggest assessing for RLS when children complain of pain in the legs, especially if there are accompanying problems with sleep.[27] Younger children may not even realize that what they're experiencing isn't normal.

To better detect whether low ferritin is a potential culprit in sleep issues, you have to look at sleep behavior and how they respond (or have responded) to sleep training efforts. Children with low ferritin levels typically do not respond *at all* to sleep training efforts. In fact, they may go a little ballistic if you even try. Many of the most intense sleep problems I've seen as a coach have been a result of low ferritin. Here are some examples:

- A three-year-old whose parents had to drive them around in the car every time they woke at night because that was the only way to get them back to sleep
- A fifteen-month-old whose mom had to stand holding them with their legs dangling from midnight until 4 or 5 AM every night
- A child who took hours to get to sleep at bedtime, woke every hour, moaned or cried in his sleep, and was awake from 2 to 4 AM almost every night
- An eight-month-old who had hourly waking even while co-sleeping and needed to sleep on top of mom with their legs dangling off the side

Low ferritin manifests as *sudden, significant,* and *immovable* problems with falling asleep and / or staying asleep (these are not just your usual bad sleep issues). Difficulties can emerge suddenly and inexplicably. Children with low ferritin can take a long time to go to sleep at bedtime and/or will be awake in the middle of the night for an hour or more. Other signs include *really* restless sleep with lots of movement, kicking, or thrashing. Parents will often notice this when they've thrown in the towel and start co-sleeping. I've had parents say that even though they were co-sleeping, the child still needed to sleep on top of or with their legs up on a parent, or they moved so much in their sleep that the parents were awake all night. Any of these symptoms by themselves may not indicate RLS. But if sleep is truly awful and there are several symptomatic behaviors happening, it's worth considering whether RLS is the issue.

Symptoms:

- Kicking, thrashing, lots of movement (at bedtime and/or when sleeping)
- Banging legs on the mattress
- Older infants and up: Wanting to stand up, refusing to lie down
- Needing to be picked up (like the mattress is lava)
- Restless and/or wakeful even when co-sleeping
- Preferring to have legs up on something / someone or have legs dangling (if you are holding them)
- Taking a long time to go to sleep, with difficulty getting comfortable
- Being awake for long periods in the middle of the night
- Older children: Complaining of pain or itchy, tickly, prickly sensations in the legs
- BIG distress in the face of sleep training attempts (lots and lots of crying with no change over time)

Risk factors:

- Mom was anemic / low iron in pregnancy
- Child has or had a food intolerance / allergy or history of reflux / silent reflux
- Family history of RLS or low iron

There's good news and bad news about low ferritin. The bad news is that proper diagnosis involves a blood draw (not a finger stick), so it can sometimes be tricky to get a pediatrician to authorize it. The good news is that treatment is just prescription-level iron supplementation (a multivitamin with iron typically isn't enough to make a dent in low levels). If you *do* get your child tested, always ask for the exact number. From a sleep medicine perspective, the threshold for needing supplementation is much higher than the cutoff that pediatricians use. You can also consult with a local children's hospital sleep clinic to get an assessment of whether your child needs iron supplementation. While it can take several months of supplementation for iron levels to come back up, sleep should start improving well before that point.

Lingering reflux / silent reflux

Though reflux / silent reflux typically resolves on its own by the time a child is sitting and/or starting solids, symptoms can linger after you think that they should have subsided. Even if you think their reflux went away a while ago, if your older baby or toddler is still persistently fussy and has any of the symptoms (page 71 for these), it's something to consider. Check with your pediatrician.

Food allergy, intolerance, or sensitivity

Food allergies / sensitivities and food intolerance are systemic reactions to substances in certain foods, and they can provoke a range of physiological responses that can absolutely affect sleep.

Food allergies / sensitivities tend to trigger clear allergic reactions, like hives, diarrhea, or other symptoms. Food *intolerances*, on the other hand, can be harder to pin down because their symptoms are less obvious. But both of these (mostly genetic) vulnerabilities can be tested with a simple finger prick.[28]

If your livewire is chronically fussy or wakeful, has frequent illnesses, or has skin issues like eczema—and no other causes appear to be the culprit—food intolerance may be something to consider. In one study in the UK, thirteen-month-olds with persistent and unexplained sleep issues who were taken off all dairy products had their sleep improve dramatically.[29]

Dairy intolerance / sensitivity (which includes the full spectrum of dairy products) is one of the most common intolerances. Other common intolerances include potato, sugar, honey, gluten, eggs, nuts, soy, fish, and citrus.[30] These substances do not have to be consumed directly to be problematic. Allergens can be transmitted through breast milk or in formula. If you yourself have food-related sensitivities, it's possible that your child does, too. Check with your pediatrician or a licensed naturopath if you are concerned.

Symptoms:
- Eczema (see the symptoms that follow)
- Gassiness / digestive issues
- Constipation or blood in the stool
- Dark circles under the eyes

Eczema (atopic dermatitis)

Eczema is a skin condition that involves itchy patches, often on the joints but on other parts of the body or face as well. Livewires, for some reason, seem prone to it—so much so that, in my coaching, when I hear that a child has eczema, I think, *Ding, ding, ding! Livewire.* It's like their entire system is more reactive and sensitive, skin included. Eczema is usually a marker for underlying food-related issues. In fact, one study found that children with eczema were six times more likely to have a food sensitivity.[31]

While eczema is not a "serious" condition, it can cause a significant level of itchiness that is known to disrupt sleep all by itself.[32] Even when parents use creams or block children from scratching, the itch may still be there. As one doctor told Kim, eczema is "the itch that rashes"—meaning your child could be itchy before patches even appear. Remember that just about *any* amount of discomfort is going to distract a livewire from sleep. It takes so much less sensation to throw a livewire off the go-to-sleep train. An itchy livewire will not be a sleeping livewire.

Feeding issues

Problems with feeding during the day (e.g., food refusal) can result in an overhungry kiddo during the night. This is true for toddlers and preschoolers, as well as infants.

Sensitive livewires can have oral processing sensitivities that impact their desire to eat many foods. An occupational therapist, feeding specialist, or myofunctional therapist can help you assess the issue and give you strategies to help.

If you are concerned about your baby or toddler's food intake, be sure to get it checked before you start working on sleep. We really don't want you worried that your child is hungry in the middle of the night. That nagging fear of *"What if they're hungry?"* can cause doubt and inconsistency, and we want you to be confident that there's nothing standing in the way of you working on your livewire's sleep skills.

Symptoms:

- Not gaining weight well
- Persistent gas or constipation
- Crying while nursing
- Taking a very long time to eat (more than thirty minutes)
- Arching back or stiffening when feeding (also may indicate tongue / lip tie)
- After eight months: Refusing purees
- Once eating solids: Refusing foods with certain textures

Musculoskeletal issues (tightness, misalignment, etc.)

If your child is a little late on any of the motor milestones or you've noticed really anything different about their movement (*"They can roll, but they just don't want to"* or *"My baby just screams / gets exhausted during tummy time"*), you may want to get an assessment. Physical therapy is sometimes prescribed if babies have difficulty with weakness / low muscle tone, tight muscles, or torticollis.

Infants can also have issues of tightness or misalignment from the birth process or even because of silent reflux and colic. These issues are often difficult to figure out because . . . well, the baby can't tell us. Sleep issues can be a good indicator. We don't think of small infants as having muscle soreness or other kinds of body-related issues, but they can. Lying in one position (like they do before they're really mobile) can cause muscles to tighten up. If you feel like your baby is waking because they seem uncomfortable and/or you also notice anything "off" in their motor skills, consult a professional.

Craniosacral therapy is a gentle intervention that can work to relieve any pain that may be affecting a baby's ability to relax and sleep. Pediatric or infant chiropractic works similarly. Both have been shown to reduce discomfort and improve sleep.[33] The nice thing about these interventions is that you may only need one or two sessions. It's an easy thing to try. Make sure, however, that you look for practitioners that have training in working with infants.

Symptoms:

- Late on some motor milestones
- Physical asymmetry (one side looks or behaves differently: one arm is weaker, child won't look to one side, etc.)
- Some tasks appear to be hard and/or painful

Obstructed breathing / apnea

Children's tonsils and adenoids can grow disproportionately to their skull, and enlarged glands can block breathing and make sleep incredibly difficult. If your child's sleep is really fractured and they have one or more of the symptoms that follow, check with a pediatric ear, nose, and throat (ENT) doctor to get their tonsils and adenoids checked. With younger children (those under three), doctors will often want to wait to see if growth patterns even out or if the breathing issues are due to allergies or other causes. For older children, they may recommend a sleep study and/or surgery to help improve breathing. If the following symptoms sound like your child, it's always good to get them checked, regardless of age.

This is also where an oral facial myofunctional therapist can be instrumental. They are trained to assess many factors of a child's health and history, including their breathing and feeding, and to identify tongue and lip ties to overall help correct mouth-breathing patterns that may not be related to enlarged glands. Poor breathing during sleep can lead to less oxygen in the body, poor growth and development, and more fractured sleep patterns.

Symptoms:

- Restless sleep
- Snoring or breathing through their mouth (outside of having a cold)
- Sweaty head while sleeping
- Frequent ear infections
- Older child: Awakening afraid at night

BEFORE MOVING FORWARD

If any of these sound like your livewire, it's critical to get the issue checked out and addressed before you even start working on sleep. Livewires are already such sensitive sleepers that if you add even a little physical discomfort to the mix, you are going to have tons more struggle. It's also important to be as sure as you can that nothing else is going on. We really want you to feel free of any nagging doubts that can be addressed before you start.

OUR TRIP CHECKLIST

- ☑ You know you are on a different path.
- ☑ You understand your livewire's temperament strengths and challenges.
- ☑ You understand the link between temperament and sleep issues.

☑ **Your child is ready:**
- **Over six months**
- **No upcoming disruptions**
- **No physiological issues that affect sleep**

☐ You are ready (or as ready as you can be).

☐ You understand the Big Four sources of sleep issues.

☐ Big Strategy #1: You know how to avoid that second wind.

☐ Big Strategy #2: You have a solid, consistent bedtime routine.

☐ Big Strategy #3 and #4: You know how to change the go-to-sleep and back-to-sleep patterns and are prepared to be more consistent than you've ever been before.

☐ You know how to track progress.

☐ You know how to diagnose and fix any problems that arise.

☐ BETTER SLEEP!

CHAPTER 5

Are You Ready?

(Or as Ready as You Can Be)

All right, we've made sure that your child is ready for working on new sleep patterns. Now we also need to make sure that *you* are ready to climb this hill.

We can't just charge in and start talking about sleep strategies. We know it's not that simple. First, by the time parents of livewires reach out for help with sleep, they are often like the walking dead. Their tanks are hovering on empty, and they feel like shell-shocked roadkill. If this is you, don't worry, we are going to move forward with all of that firmly in mind. We want to structure our approach so that we don't overwhelm anyone involved—including you.

Second, you may be worried about poking this particular bear.

> *It's possible that you've muscled your livewire's
> sleep to a place where it's at least not a
> nightmare, and you're worried that if you do
> anything differently, you could make it worse.*

Or maybe you're worried about how this might affect your livewire (*"Can they handle it? Will it wreck your relationship with them? Will it even work?"*).

Ambivalence about tackling sleep issues is unbelievably common when you have a livewire. I mean, who can blame you? The prospect of trying to change the status quo may feel like you're just asking for trouble. I've seen so many parents who are really struggling but are also terrified of attempting to change things because they know what they could be in for. I get it. I really do. (I mean, this is exactly why I didn't try sleep training.)

Here are some important points to consider that may help you get some clarity:

REALITY CHECK #1: Is the status quo sustainable? If you have figured out a way to make sleep tolerable for now, that's great. But it's so important to ask yourself: Is it sustainable? Can you continue lying on the floor for an hour in the dark with your hand up in the crib for much longer? Even if co-sleeping is mostly working now, will it still be okay with you in six months? Two years? (Will your partner *ever* be able to come back into your room?)

REALITY CHECK #2: Sleep won't get better on its own. Lots of livewire parents are doing their best to just hang in there and avoid actively sleep training because they think (hope), *It could resolve on its own any day now, and then I don't have to even worry about sleep training* (this was totally me). Mayyybe. But, with livewires, probably not. As a baseline, they need more help with sleep, and they are even *less* likely to just abandon their preferred sleep strategies (bouncing, nursing, parent proximity, etc.). Some experts will tell you that if you just follow your baby's cues, they will gradually learn to sleep on their own and just naturally drop those middle-of-the-night feeds. Real talk? If this ever happens with livewires, I haven't seen it. Once they have a pattern that works and that they're comfortable with, why would they drop it? Why would they think there's a different way to do it? These patterns almost always need a pretty definitive nudge.

If you *know* you can't keep going with the status quo, but you're worried about how changing it could impact your child, let me reassure you:

1. We're going to make *sure* that whatever we are asking of your live-wire is completely in their wheelhouse.
2. When you are so tired you can barely function, it is okay to ask your little ball of fire to bend a little and learn some new skills.

Livewires require *a lot* from their parents. To keep up with them, we need brain cells, patience, and stamina. If you are trying to keep up with your livewire on paltry shreds of sleep, you have none of these. Over time, the consequences of chronic exhaustion are no joke (we'll talk more about it in chapter fourteen).

Some parents feel very hesitant about trying to push their livewire. I get that. On the other hand, I can tell you from experience that sacrificing your health because you don't want to ask your livewire to stretch a little and learn a few sleep skills is not a good way to go. It's okay to ask them to meet you a little in the middle, so they get the sleep they need and you can keep body and soul together. You need all the energy you can get just to keep up with them in the daytime. There may be a temporary bit of struggle but the payoff is going to be huge.

Whether you're dealing with a couple of stubborn trouble spots or sleep in your house needs a complete down-to-the-studs overhaul, here's another promise: We're not going to require you to do anything you don't feel ready for. Parents who feel pushed to do something they don't want to do or that goes against their instincts are more likely to bail too early. Or ambivalence about the method makes their responses so inconsistent or unclear that there's no progress, and they give up. You have to feel *ready* to tackle the road ahead and confident that whatever you decide to do for sleep is tolerable for you, your livewire, and your family.

CHECKING UNDER *YOUR* HOOD

So, maybe you aren't in full burnout yet. That's good. Let's take a moment, though, to assess your energy level.

Are you running on fumes?

Most livewire parents are more exhausted than any human should be. The thought that their situation could get any harder just doesn't seem physically possible. I've had parents tell me, "I honestly can't handle 'harder.'" When sleep has been bad for a long time, some parents are so completely depleted (both from lack of sleep and from the extra energy livewires require all day long) that there's really nothing left in their tank, and parts of their engine are grinding and smoking. If you are raising your hand, saying, "This is me," I know you are starting from a rough place. There is a good-size push that needs to be made at the beginning of this process, and you need to have at least a little bandwidth to be able to make it.

What you can do when you're this tired:

Put at least a *little* gas in your tank before you start working on sleep skills. Have the grandparents come over for a night while the parents go to a hotel, hire a night doula / nurse, or get a friend to take the baby for several hours while you take a nap (with earplugs). Get a little bit of sleep so that you are going into sleep work with a clearer head.

Pick one thing. You can absolutely go slower and potentially just pick *one* sleep issue to work on. Here's the catch: You have to be really committed to that one task. For example, you can *just* work on bedtime skills and do whatever you've been doing for the rest of the night. Or you can work on swapping one soothing strategy for a new one (instead of nursing to sleep, you bounce on a ball to sleep instead). Choosing just one goal can make the process feel manageable. It also can give you a teeny taste of progress, which is sometimes all that's necessary to give you enough confidence and encouragement to do more.

Share the load. Working on sleep can be a great time for partners to step up by taking the lead on establishing a new go-to-sleep routine. This is especially true when one partner is nursing, and you're going to lay down a new, non-nursing-dependent sleeping pattern. This can work like magic because, chances are, the non-nursing partner is not quite as pooped, and your livewire gets the message: new person, new plan. Since that partner also *can't* nurse, it's easier for the child to recognize that feeding to sleep is not gonna happen. There will still be protest, but the way forward may be clearer once nursing is no longer an option.

Is your emotional engine overheating a lot?

Non-sleeping livewires can be the source of high levels of parental frustration, hopelessness, and anger. A three-year-old who is out of bed for the twelfth time since lights out is going to drive just about anyone around the bend. Mix in a heaping helping of livewire bedtime (and daytime) meltdowns, and you could be ready to jump out of your own skin.

There are times when we truly get ground down to a powder with how hard this path can be. Sometimes, for a variety of reasons, we arrive at a place where we dread the person we become when bedtime rolls around. This may be especially true for parents who have a history of trauma or issues from childhood, or who are *also* livewires. But really, it can be true for *anyone* parenting a livewire.

If you feel that things have reached a boiling point and everything feels frustrating or gets under your skin—if you feel like you're yelling a lot (it totally happens)—this may not be the right time to start sleep coaching. If *you* aren't able to be grounded and somewhat emotionally regulated, your child won't be able to, either. We can't teach self-soothing from a place of internal freak-out. Without some bit of internal okay-ness, you *definitely* won't be able to navigate those harder first days of working on sleep.

What you can do when you feel chronically triggered:

Take the pot off the boil. You will not be able to think straight if your emotions are running high. To bring stress levels down to a more manageable level, take a step back and do whatever works for sleep, just for a bit, so that tensions can subside. That may mean that for a few days you let your child sleep in your room all night or you camp out in their room. This is a short-term bandage so everyone can get a few full nights of sleep, and everyone can reset. There is nothing wrong with doing what works for the short-term, resetting, and starting again once you don't feel like you're boiling over every five minutes.

Commit to some self-calming and self-care. If your gas tank is empty or you're really feeling triggered, you're not going to be able to help anyone. I know it sounds impossible and like I'm giving you the "just take a bubble bath" speech, but trust me—try to give yourself some grace, some education on self-calming strategies, and a teeny tiny break. See chapter fourteen for more on this.

PRE-TRIP JITTERS

So, your livewire is ready, and maybe *you* are even ready (sort of), but there are still a few more (totally common) nagging worries that put *just* that little bit of doubt into the mix. Let's get those out of the way.

"I'm worried about how much crying there might be." (Or "How bad is 'bad'?")

I know, I know. It's already pretty bad, and you're nervous about the possibility of "worse." Real talk: The first couple of times that you introduce a change in familiar sleep patterns, it's going to be a rodeo. What does that mean in actual *amounts* of struggle? In our experience, ninety minutes is usually on the upper end of "bad." It could be a little longer. It could also be less. (You *literally* never know with these unpredictable ones.) It's going to depend on a lot of different factors: your child's age, how many methods you've already tried, what's going on at home, etc.

But here's a big idea that we want you to remember:

We're not going to leave your livewire to cry
by themselves, and you will always be able to
help them calm down when they need it.

We're not going to let anyone get hysterical and then just leave them like that. You will be there with them: supporting, encouraging, monitoring, helping them calm down when you feel like they need it. We're going to do everything possible to set both of you up for success. We are going to make absolutely sure that what you are planning to tackle is in their wheelhouse and yours. In this context, crying will not be about fear or abandonment. They will have you *right there* physically and emotionally. So, then, we have to ask: What else could the crying be about? It's more likely that they've noticed (and strongly dislike) the change you've made and are really confused about what the heck you are doing or expecting them to do. We can't explain it to them ahead of time. So, from their perspective, we've just thrown them a curveball, and they're trying to get the situation to go back to how it was before. As parents, we can empathize with their frustration and still keep moving forward.

Here's the other critical piece: You get to pick them up to calm them down as soon as you think they need it. We're going to help them hold that heavy bag. The kind of crying we worry about (the kind that raises cortisol a lot) comes from overwhelming distress that goes on for a long time and is not co-regulated by a caregiver. Remember, we're not going to leave them alone to manage it. You're going to be there to help.

"But my livewire cries so hard, they throw up."

Some livewires are so intense that even the slightest change causes them to absolutely lose it.

"My child starts hyperventilating the minute we move toward their room."

"I've tried putting them in the crib not fully asleep and it's like the end of the world."

We've encountered some very intense livewires in our work, and, yes, they can act like the world is ending if you're not doing what you normally do. Again, don't worry. If you have one of these bottle-rocket criers, you will be able to go more slowly. There's no sense in letting anyone get so upset that they can't handle it. Both Kim and I have found in working with uber intense livewires that staying with them really short-circuits the vomiting. And in chapters nine, ten, and eleven, we're going to help you figure out the sweet spot between jumping in too soon and not jumping in soon enough.

"I'm worried that this will damage our attachment."

Parents understandably wonder whether their child's crying during sleep coaching will damage their relationship with their child. They worry that holding back soothing will cause the child to no longer trust that the parent is present and available.

Here's an important piece of information to know:

Attachment isn't that fragile.

Attachment doesn't change day to day. It gets established through a reasonably reliable and consistent pattern of response *over time*. Responses don't have to be perfect—just relatively predictable, consistent, and "good enough." Attachment style doesn't change just because one night, you didn't pick your baby up fast enough.

A secure attachment, which is always the goal, also doesn't mean that a child *never* experiences distress. A secure attachment results from parents keeping distress at a *tolerable* level and stepping in fairly consistently when they're really needed. You might be interested to know that attachment stems from not only attuned responses to distress but also moments of mismatch and reconnections. These moments of *repair* can be critical to emotional regulation and attachment.[34] Here's a typical example: The child gets upset and cries to be picked up or attended to but the parent is occupied with a task. Once the parent realizes and rejoins the baby, the baby comes back to feeling okay. Distress-response exchanges between parents and children absolutely can't (and shouldn't be) perfect.

It might surprise you that the heart and soul of attachment *isn't* just the action of soothing. It's the fact that you have *noticed* your child's signals and are *trying* to interpret them. Is your child wet? Hungry? Overtired? Bored? Frustrated? In attachment theory, this is called *mentalizing*.[35] When you work to interpret your child's cries, you are using your adult emotion processing system to interpret that signal, essentially translating your child's raw emotional communication. The way you respond to them based on that translation helps wire their emerging emotional regulation system.

Here's what this might look like from the baby's perspective:

BABY: *Waaah! Something feels baaaad!!!!*

PARENT: What's going on? Hmm . . . I wonder if you're hungry. Let me feed you.

BABY: *Ahhh. That's better. My big people get me. I exist, and all is well.*

Over time, the baby learns to equate that bodily signal with needing to eat. They learn that feeling is hunger.

Thinking about your baby's communicated signal and then responding as appropriately as you can is the beginning of emotional communication between you and your child, and *this* is the foundation of attachment. *A secure attachment does not mean that you know what to do every time your child is upset.* It just means that you are *trying*. Often, livewires have signals that are hard to decode. You may be worried that you're *not* interpreting their signals because you can't tell what the heck they're signaling. They *don't* calm down, even though you've tried a bunch of things. What if you've consistently gotten it wrong? Well, first, you haven't always gotten it wrong, I promise. Second, you are *trying* to puzzle out what's going on, and *that's* the important piece.

Insecure attachment comes from *chronic* patterns of misinterpreting a child's signals and/or responding inappropriately to their signal: too little (or no) response, wrong response, incomplete response, unpredictable response—even *way too much* response. It can't be emphasized enough that attachment is about an *overarching* pattern, not day-to-day or moment-by-moment events.

"I'm still worried that crying will damage them."

I know you may still be worried about what could happen the first time you don't do what you usually do at bedtime. When we change the status quo and disrupt what a livewire expects to happen, they are going to cry. *However*, our approach is not like the other methods. Most sleep strategies involve you leaving the room and allowing only brief pop-ins for a little bit of soothing; you are not allowed to stay long or pick them up. This is *very* different from what we're going to propose. You get to stay in the room, providing lots of support and picking them up to calm them down *as soon as* you think they need help. There are no timers and no rules about what you can or can't do. You get to keep your livewire inside their window of tolerance.

> **A child's window of tolerance is how much distress they can capably handle for not only their age but also their temperament.**

As we discussed in chapter four, children have capacities for managing distress that grow as they age. Over time, they develop a wider array of skills. The older the child, the more options they have for self-soothing. But children of any age can need help getting back down to calm—or at least a more manageable level—when distress becomes more intense than they can manage. Once distress is tolerable again, children can start to use some of those self-soothing tricks. When it's not manageable, they need help from you. Remember the heavy bag analogy? Livewires experience more feeling at a faster rate and so their window of tolerance is smaller than it is for dandelions. For livewires, almost *everything* weighs a hundred pounds, and they need help reducing the load.

It's also important to know that while we don't want to *over*challenge livewires, we also don't want to *under*challenge them. If we never give them bits of frustration to practice with, they don't get a chance to develop strategies they can use to deal with it. The trick is to figure out the size of their window so that we are giving support when it's needed but also allowing them to wrestle with a little frustration that can ultimately help them learn new skills.

> **The other important point here is that crying in the presence of a supportive, loving parent is fundamentally different from crying alone in a room.**

Douglas Teti and colleagues at the University of Pennsylvania have done some amazing work on the role of parents' emotional availability at bedtime and its effects on both cortisol (the stress hormone) and sleep. *Emotional availability* means that the parent is emotionally present with their child while helping them learn sleep skills. The research found that emotional availability at bedtime significantly reduced the child's (and parent's) stress levels and resulted in much better sleep overall.[36] Being emotionally and physically available to your child while you work on sleep is qualitatively different from leaving the room—even when your child ends up crying while you're there.

"I'm worried that my child will feel ignored or like I don't love them."

I get this worry. But, just like attachment, your relationship isn't this fragile. You have likely done a million things to communicate to your child that you are there, ready, and willing to love them through whatever life brings.

We can't possibly give our children everything in this life that they want. There will be many, many times when you are going to have to say no. You know this. Asking them to bend a little so that their nights and yours are more manageable is not an unreasonable request. Be confident that you've built a boatload of trust with your livewire. You can't undo it just because they're outraged that you're changing things up.

If we can also go a little deeper for just a brief moment: As parents, we all have *stuff* from our own childhoods. We may not even know it's there until we have babies of our own, and then—*bam!*—*stuff* erupts out of nowhere, especially when you are sleep-deprived. Going to sleep at night is a big separation for both baby *and* parent. We may have complex feelings about this. Trying to work on sleep can poke at some of our own buried attachment injuries.

When we interpret our baby's crying, there's a difference between trying to figure out what they need (*mentalizing*) and *projection*, where we attribute to our child *our* experiences as children. How do you know the difference? Carefully observe what you say to yourself.

If you say things like "They're feeling so abandoned" or "They think I don't care," pay attention.

Ask yourself whether this is really what your child is feeling or a buried remnant from your own childhood (for example, *"When I was a child, I was alone a lot and I felt so abandoned. I don't want my baby to feel that way, too"*). Emotional buttons can get pushed hard when it *feels* like you're putting your baby in the same situation.

It's important to remember that your livewire is having a different childhood than you did. Their experience is not the same as yours because they have *you* as a parent. You are doing the hard work of not only healing yourself but also stopping the transmission of dysfunctional patterns. It's not easy work, but boy, is it important. From time to time as you move forward in working on sleep, check in with yourself. Pay attention to those ouchy spots and validate them, but also know that you are giving your child a different experience than the one you had (yay, you!).

"I'm worried that, emotionally, I just won't be able to do it."

This is a really valid concern. Sensitive, intense livewires often have sensitive, intense parents for whom crying sets off every alarm bell they have.

Plus, parents are *wired* to respond to a crying child. It's totally normal (and a great gift) to be this tuned in to your child.

I wish there were a way to make this sleep-improvement process completely no cry, but there isn't. We can't make changes that a livewire won't notice. I can promise you, though, that we build in lots of preparation and groundwork so that we avoid freaking them out unnecessarily.

Here's something I also want you to consider: It's *really easy* to get into a trap of overresponding to a livewire when they react like the world is ending. Sensitive parents hear those intense cries and think, *Good grief! They're really afraid / sad / in pain*. It's possible that they're not as afraid / sad / in pain as they sound, and they're just expressing themselves *strongly* (like livewires do). Sensitive parents sometimes need a little practice allowing their child to have those *manageable* bits of frustration. If we are present and supportive, livewires will be okay even when they're a little freaked out. Take it from two moms of young adults: When they ultimately hit adolescence, you will need to be okay with them losing it when you say no to something they want to do. *Practice now.*

"My partner and I don't really agree on how to approach sleep training."

Disagreement over sleep training strategies can be a huge source of couple conflict that is only exacerbated by fatigue. Conflicting ideas about parenting philosophy or what sleep training method to use can throw a massive monkey wrench into the process (we've seen it happen). With sensitive, perceptive livewires, it is especially important to agree on the path forward because inconsistency (or outright conflict) is going to be a progress killer. Here's the good news: Because the approach we're going to use represents a middle ground between following cues until the end of time and full-on crying it out, it has a ton of room for compromise. There should be a way to craft an effective strategy that both partners feel okay about.

Before you begin to work on sleep, we encourage you to have some solid discussion about how you both want to proceed. It's important to

be honest. This is the moment to really discuss feelings around sleep and
identify any big disconnects. How much work will each partner be able to
do? How well can they hang in there when the child is losing it on the first
night? Do your best to understand where you are on the same page and
where you're not.

If disagreements ultimately have more to do with underlying relationship issues than disagreements about sleep training, use this as an
opportunity to seek out some help. Becoming parents is no joke. Having a
non-sleeping livewire can add to that stress. Get support and intervention
from a caring professional if you can. Perceptive little livewires pick up on
and react to *everything*. As much as possible, try to build a team mentality
around working on sleep.

If one parent truly can't participate (health reasons, travel, etc.) or
won't, that parent at least needs to agree that they will support the parent
doing the work. Even better, they can agree to take the baby / child in the
morning, so the partner who's sleep coaching gets some sleep.

"I'm divorced / single / widowed / my partner is deployed."

First of all, you are working so hard. This is still doable for you, but it's also
okay to go as slowly as you need to and make sure you take care of your own
mental health. You are on deck 24-7, and you only have a certain amount
of energy.

In chapter ten, we'll cover ways to break this process into manageable pieces. If you are a single parent, see if you can wrangle some extra
support (especially if you have another child / other children). If you are
co-parenting, know that children can understand different sets of rules. It's
of course better if both places are using the same approach, but if that's not
possible, it's okay. Whatever your solo situation is, proceed as slowly as you
need to go.

GREEN LIGHT: READY TO ROCK AND ROLL

Now that we've made sure everyone is ready, it's time to get a handle on where you're starting from, how far you need to go, and what it's going to take to get there. Time to pack the car and get ready to hit the road.

OUR TRIP CHECKLIST

- ☑ You know you are on a different path.
- ☑ You understand your livewire's temperament strengths and challenges.
- ☑ You understand the link between temperament and sleep issues.
- ☑ Your child is ready:
    - ☑ Over six months
    - ☑ No upcoming disruptions
    - ☑ No physiological issues that affect sleep
- ☑ You are ready (or as ready as you can be).
- ☐ You understand the Big Four sources of sleep issues.
- ☐ Big Strategy #1: You know how to avoid that second wind.
- ☐ Big Strategy #2: You have a solid, consistent bedtime routine.
- ☐ Big Strategy #3 and #4: You know how to change the go-to-sleep and back-to-sleep patterns and are prepared to be more consistent than you've ever been before.
- ☐ You know how to track progress.
- ☐ You know how to diagnose and fix any problems that arise.
- ☐ BETTER SLEEP!

Charting a New Course

CHAPTER 6

The Big Four Sleep Tankers and How to Tackle Them

We have officially laid a solid foundation of preparation for where we need to go:

- You know about your livewire's temperament: check.
- You've ruled out anything that could stand in the way of improvement: check.
- You feel ready to go (mostly): check.

We're now going to look at the struggles you are having (and have had in the past) with sleep. The really great news? Most of these problems boil down to *just four issues* that will become the focus of your new approach to finally fixing your livewire's lack of sleep. If you are like most (yes, *most*—or even *all*) parents of livewires, you probably have a long list of sleep issues that you want to tackle (unless there's a choice that's just "all of the above"). In my research, I found that parents of livewires had longer lists of sleep problems and less success with the methods they had already tried to fix them. So, you are not alone if you check a lot of the following boxes.

Right now, your livewire . . .

☐ Wakes up for the day before 6 AM.

☐ Won't go to sleep until 9 or 10 PM.

☐ Will not nap and/or takes naps that are super short.

☐ Takes a million years to go to sleep at bedtime (not at all sleepy).

☐ Takes a million years to go to sleep at bedtime (meltdowns, stalling, shenanigans).

☐ Needs feeding / rocking / holding / physical contact at bedtime and/or during the night.

☐ Goes to sleep well but wakes frequently.

☐ Doesn't go to sleep well and wakes frequently.

☐ Goes to sleep well but is up for an hour or more during the night.

☐ Won't stay in their bed.

☐ Is still co-sleeping / still in your room.

☐ Starts out in their room / crib but ends up in your bed.

☐ Needs a parent to sleep in their room every night.

Here's some amazing news: For livewires, most of these problems stem from what I call:

THE BIG FOUR SLEEP TANKERS

#1 Overtiredness

#2 Problems with the lead-up to lights out (transitions and routine)

#3 Parent is a required part of the go-to-sleep and back-to-sleep pattern

#4 Past inconsistency (trying a method, then stopping too soon or only partly trying)

Believe it or not, the Big Four are behind almost *all* of the common sleep challenges. See the following table for examples. (Don't worry, we'll explain all of these in detail later.)

Problem	Potential culprit	Tanker
Up before 6 AM	Too little naptime	#1 Overtired
	Too late a bedtime	#1 Overtired
	One or more wake windows that are too long	#1 Overtired
	Being too drowsy at bedtime (being put in bed almost or fully asleep)	#2 Lead-up to lights out #3 Parent is part of the pattern
Won't go to sleep until 9 or 10 PM	Too little naptime	#1 Overtired
	Too late a bedtime	#1 Overtired
	Inconsistent routine, not enough wind down	#2 Lead-up to lights out #4 Past inconsistency
Bedtime takes a million years	Too little naptime	#1 Overtired
	Too late a bedtime	#1 Overtired
	Needs more transition and wind down	#2 Lead-up to lights out
Goes to sleep well but wakes frequently	Too little naptime	#1 Overtired
	Being too drowsy at bedtime (fell asleep too fast)	#2 Lead-up to lights out
	Being fed / rocked to sleep	#3 Parent is part of the pattern
Doesn't go to sleep well and wakes frequently	Too little naptime	#1 Overtired
	Too late a bedtime	#1 Overtired
	Being fed / rocked to sleep	#3 Parent is part of the pattern

Here's more good news: While the Big Four represent where sleep can veer off the rails, they are *also* how we get everything back on track. We are going to focus most of our energy on strategies that target these four trouble spots so that you can improve your livewire's sleep once and for all (or at least until the next regression, vacation, or illness).

BIG STRATEGY #1: AVOID THE DREADED OVERTIRED / WIRED SECOND WIND

Working on the timing and amount of sleep is one of the *easiest* and *most influential* actions we can take to improve all aspects of sleep—especially for livewires. Yes, I'm serious. Livewires have a strong drive to stay awake and keep engaging in the world. They have nonexistent sleepy signals and get a massive burst of energy if you don't get them to sleep in that micro-moment when they might be ready.

I've heard parents say, "But they're just not tired until 10 PM." They *are* tired, but because they have stayed awake past the point where they needed to go to sleep, they are now fully into their second wind. Overtiredness can cause a host of problems: bedtime struggles, more night waking, and even earlier morning wake-ups. Missing that sleep window means that *all* sleep is harder.

Livewires don't get tired; they get wired.

Simply adjusting the timing of sleep so that you stay in front of the second wind can, all by itself, significantly improve both daytime and nighttime sleep.

A strategy that's easy *and* impactful? Yes, please.

We'll talk more about this in chapter seven.

BIG STRATEGY #2: HAVE AN EFFECTIVE LEAD-UP TO LIGHTS OUT

How you transition an active, busy livewire into bedtime really matters, so we're going to be talking about leveling up the bedtime routine you currently have in place. Having a well-planned routine (and even a *pre-routine* routine) gives livewires enough lead-up time and a reliable structure so they can better navigate the turn from go, go, go to bedtime.

For non-livewires, a quick bath, book, and song may be all that's necessary for them to be ready for shut-eye. I'm willing to bet that your bedtime doesn't look anything like this. Livewire bedtimes can be a full three-ring circus. With babies, it can be marathon bouncing or nursing sessions. For older kiddos, lots of books and a million "one last things" and then lying with them for hours while they struggle to fall asleep. The bedtime drama won't be *solved* just by changing up the routine, but a more structured bedtime, with actions and activities that signal bedtime is coming, can make the whole lights-out process a little more manageable.

In chapter eight, we're going to fold in some of those pre-routine activities. Then we're going to look at sensory strategies that will help your livewire physically and mentally calm down. For older livewires (two and a half years and older), crafting a set-in-stone Bedtime Chart with a predictable sequence of steps and clear limits on what will and won't happen at bedtime can be a game-changer.

BIG STRATEGY #3: SHIFT THEIR GO-TO-SLEEP (AND BACK-TO-SLEEP) PATTERN SO THAT IT INVOLVES LESS OF *YOU*

Once you've set the stage by staying ahead of their second wind and giving them lots of predictable transition time into bedtime, we're going to help your livewire learn a new way of going to sleep (and, by extension, *back* to sleep) that gradually involves less and less of *you* as part of the process.

We want to emphasize that whatever is going on now at bedtime isn't a "bad habit." The way your child is going to sleep now is just how they believe it's done. For all they know, this is how *you* go to sleep, too.

What happens *as they fall asleep* at bedtime establishes the template for how sleep happens and what they will try to re-create to get back to sleep.

"I have a bottle, and I'm rocked, and . . ."—they wake up in the crib / bed without you—*"Wait a minute, how did I get here? Helllooo?! I need that bottle and rocking thing to get back to sleep."*

Or, for an older kiddo:

"Dad is sitting beside me, and I'm holding his finger, and . . ."—when they wake and Dad's not in his chair—*"Hey, Dad! You need to come back and sit in the chair so I can hold your finger and go to sleep!"*

If *you* are part of their bedtime template, you'll be part of their middle-of-the-night template, too. We're going to talk in detail in chapters ten and eleven about how to make sure that doesn't happen anymore.

BIG STRATEGY #4: CONSISTENCY, CONSISTENCY, CONSISTENCY

We're going to ask you to be more consistent than you've ever, ever been while you work on sleep. I know that you can get so impossibly tired that you end up throwing everything but the kitchen sink at sleep problems with the hope that something—*anything*—will stick. You also may not feel super confident about the new strategies you're using or your ability to deploy them. When we're desperate and a new strategy doesn't immediately work, it's common to bail on it in favor of trying something else that might—for the love of heaven—work better. *"We tried 'pick up, put down,' and the first night, it was completely awful. So, we switched to pop-ins, but that was even worse, and we couldn't make it past that first night."*

If this has been you, don't stress. This is totally common and completely understandable. However, livewires do not respond well when patterns keep changing. Inconsistent responses or a succession of different strategies inadvertently make things *worse*, resulting in more intense pushback and a lot less improvement (if there's any at all).

Let's pretend I was going to teach you a dance, and I showed you the first four or five moves. You struggled to copy and learn them. But just as you were sort of catching on, I decided that since you hadn't really improved, I'd try a different dance altogether. You started trying to learn *those* steps, but I didn't give you enough time before I changed the dance yet again. You'd be frustrated (and I'd be the worst dance teacher ever).

Livewires love a pattern, and when you can lay one down that's clear and consistent, their livewire spidey senses will detect it. Then they can get with the program you're showing them. You just have to give them time to catch on and practice. They're not going to be good at it right away. When patterns change too much, livewires get really, really frustrated and may resist your next attempts even harder.

Having a clear, well-crafted plan will help you avoid making decisions or judgment calls out of desperation and on the fly. (Remember that night that you said yes to a fourth book because you didn't want a fight, and now you're *always* reading four books?) If there's been a lot of back and forth or starts and stops in your past sleep efforts, you may need to be consistent for even longer than you might have otherwise. But if you can hang in there, you *will* make progress. A plan that you feel good about gives you the confidence to really stick to your guns. (Stay tuned for chapters nine through eleven, where we'll help you create that plan.)

GETTING READY TO HEAD OUT

Understanding the Big Four and how to tackle them is critical to success in sleep with livewires. Other methods of sleep training—the ones that are made for dandelions—generally make a beeline straight to putting your child in bed, then tell you how not to respond when the crying begins. We're taking a different path, making sure the major pitfalls are well marked so you can avoid them.

The next three chapters will lead you through how to get from where you are now to where you'd like to be. We're going to give you lots of information and options so this work is as simple and straightforward as it can be. And remember, we're not going to throw your livewire into the deep end of the pool. We're going to let them tiptoe in at the shallow end and give them lots of support while they learn how to go to sleep without all the nursing and bouncing, and . . . well, you know.

OUR TRIP CHECKLIST

- ☑ You know you are on a different path.
- ☑ You understand your livewire's temperament strengths and challenges.
- ☑ You understand the link between temperament and sleep issues.
- ☑ Your child is ready:
  - ☑ Over six months
  - ☑ No upcoming disruptions
  - ☑ No physiological issues that affect sleep
- ☑ You are ready (or as ready as you can be).
- ☑ You understand the Big Four sources of sleep issues.
- ☐ Big Strategy #1: You know how to avoid that second wind.
- ☐ Big Strategy #2: You have a solid, consistent bedtime routine.
- ☐ Big Strategy #3 and #4: You know how to change the go-to-sleep and back-to-sleep patterns and are prepared to be more consistent than you've ever been before.
- ☐ You know how to track progress.
- ☐ You know how to diagnose and fix any problems that arise.
- ☐ BETTER SLEEP!

CHAPTER 7

Big Strategy #1: Avoid the Dreaded Second Wind

Sleep Timing Is Everything

Let's talk about the easiest piece of the improving-sleep puzzle: *avoiding your livewire's uber powerful second wind* by getting them enough rest at the right times. You know how it usually goes: You've missed their usual nap-time by twenty minutes, and now they're all systems go, go, go. That nap isn't *easier* because they're tired; it's harder, or even impossible.

One of the main ways that we will be laying the foundation for success at bedtime and nighttime is by staying ahead of that burst of wired, buzzy alertness.

We're going to do this by:

1. Trying for naps within the limits of their awake windows.

2. Getting them as close as we can to their daily nap / Quiet Time (page 115) targets.

3. Making sure we get them in bed at bedtime *before* they hit that second wind.

Stick with us. This will all make sense in a minute.

AVOIDING THE DAYTIME SECOND WIND: THE IMPORTANCE OF NAP TIMING AND AMOUNT

When livewires don't get enough naptime, their brains are cranking away for longer than they should without a break. (If your livewire is old enough to have successfully dropped naps, feel free to skip to page 112 on avoiding the bedtime second wind.) Children's brains need time to file the learning they are doing and reset.[37] Think of your livewire's brain as a little bucket that gets filled up with experiences and thoughts and images. To properly digest all that learning and then keep going, their bucket needs to be emptied from time to time.

Livewires tend to fill their buckets up faster because their high engagement and low sensory thresholds mean they take in more input at a time. Their brains and bodies may need a time-out sooner—even when they don't *act* like they do. And if they *don't* get a break when that bucket is full, it's like their brain goes *"Okay! I guess we're staying awake!"* and sends out a biochemical cup of coffee to keep them going. They blow right past their tired / ready-for-a-nap micromoment into the overtired / wired / no-way-I'm-sleeping-now zone, which can make sleep more difficult not just at that nap but *for the rest of the day and night.*

> *Too much awake time and/or too little naptime can directly cause more drama at bedtime, more night waking, and pesky early rising the next morning.*

Here's why that happens. Humans, regardless of age, have a biological need for rest in a twenty-four-hour period. The younger the human, the more frequently they need it. If we blow past the time when our body needs a break, chemicals like cortisol and adrenaline get released to help us stay awake.[38] It's an adaptive response. Thousands of years ago, it would not have been safe to just nod off when there were predators around. The body needs to be able to keep itself going, so it releases these compounds. It's a lot like drinking coffee when you're feeling tired. It helps you in the short-term, but if you drink it at the wrong time or have too much of it, you won't be able to go to sleep even when you want to.

Trying for a nap or Quiet Time with your livewire at the right intervals during the day is one of the easiest steps you can take to improve their sleep. You may be amazed at the progress you can make on sleep simply by getting ahead of the second wind. A well-rested livewire puts you that much farther ahead on shifting bedtime sleep patterns—simply because they aren't cranky-pants overtired.

Before you freak out . . .

Don't worry. We're not going to work on independent naps just yet. (We'll talk about nap coaching strategies in chapters ten and eleven.) While you're working on nighttime sleep skills, you want to get your livewire close to their nap targets in any way you can.

Yes, you read that right:

> **While you're working on nighttime sleep,**
> **get enough naptime in any way you can**
> **(stroller, contact, rocking, etc.).**

I know that you are probably *more than ready* for your livewire to be put down easily for their nap in their crib or bed and not on you. But we need to get their nighttime go-to-sleep skills down *first*.

Here's why. Bedtime is the *easiest and most influential time* for learning new, more independent go-to-sleep skills. The biological drive for sleep results from a release of melatonin by the brain in the early evening and sleep pressure that builds and prepares the body for sleep. You don't have that at naptime. At bedtime, you are awake and alert and your child's biochemistry gives them a head start on sleep. All of this gives a little boost to your work on sleep.

Remember, bedtime also sets your child's go-to-sleep template for both day and night. Trying to work on naps or middle-of-the-night waking *before* having a new go-to-sleep map firmly in place means you could be swimming hard upstream. Your livewire first needs to be a champ at *going to sleep* independently at bedtime, then *back to sleep* at nighttime wake-ups, and *then* we can ask them to learn new daytime go-to-sleep skills. Napping for livewires is hard enough. You really want them to have mastered go-to-sleep skills at bedtime first before you try it during the day.

Getting naps however you can is a *short-term* strategy so that you have a reasonably well-rested (not overtired) livewire when you're trying to work on bedtime skills. If you try to work on naps *and* bedtime at the same time, it's possible you could struggle throughout the day, get less naptime overall, and have an overtired, cranky kiddo for your work on bedtime. No fun. *For now*, get naps at the right time in whatever way will work. Trust me, once your livewire is a rock star at night, tackling naps will be easier. (Okay, real talk, who are we kidding? Naps for livewires may never be "easy." But if you can get good nights, at least you'll be better rested from all that nighttime sleep, and you'll be more up to the challenge.)

AVOIDING THE BEDTIME SECOND WIND: THE MAGIC OF AN EARLY BEDTIME

Getting well-timed naps not only helps you avoid the wired zone but also sets you up for a good, early bedtime. Around sunset or just after, the body starts to prepare itself for sleep: Body temperature starts to drop, there's that internal release of melatonin, and sleep pressure has built up enough that your always-active livewire is more ready for sleep than at any other point in the day. If you can jump on that little (probably microscopic) lull in energy, sleep may be much easier to get.

It's extremely common—almost par for the course—for parents to say that, although they put them to bed earlier, their livewire just doesn't seem able to fall asleep before 10 PM. This is generally because bedtime wasn't

DOES BEDTIME *HAVE* TO BE EARLY?

Is it possible to have a later bedtime? Sure. As long as you have a later wake-up, too. Noted sleep researcher Marie-Hélène Pennestri of McGill University in Montreal says, "What is more important is total sleep duration and consistency of the bedtime timing. So, is everyone able to sleep long enough?"[39] Meaning, if your child doesn't go to bed until 10 PM, do they actually sleep in until 9 or 10 AM the next day? Are you able to keep that timing roughly the same, day to day? As long as you can maintain a fairly consistent schedule that allows for enough sleep, you can decide when bedtime or wake-up time is.

early *enough*. Parents are either waiting for sleepy cues (that will never come) or trying for bed only after the second wind has already kicked in. Or they let their little one sleep in too late in the morning. A late start can mean late naps and a late bedtime. Getting your livewire in bed early can help you stay ahead of the wired zone and ensures that they're getting as much nighttime sleep as they should. (Plus, an earlier bedtime may mean a few hours of actual grown-up time for you.)

> *When you're working on adjusting your livewire's sleep schedule, always start with the shorter end of a wake window target. Then you can expand from there, experimenting to find your livewire's unique sweet spot.*

Pay attention to wake windows and always try for that earlier bedtime at first. If that time really doesn't work, try fifteen minutes later than that. Keep testing to see if there's a window where your little one falls asleep a little faster and/or sleeps a little better. Remember, livewires won't *tell* you that they're tired. You have to *assume* that they're tired, despite how alert they seem, and try to get ahead of that rocket-booster second wind.

NAP AND AWAKE WINDOW TARGETS

We're going to look at some *targets* for naps, awake windows, and night-time sleep so that you know what to shoot for. Notice that we're using the word *targets* and not *requirements*. These numbers are a place to start. Your unique child may be a little under or a little over these targets. This just gives us something to aim for initially.

First, let's look at the timing and amount of sleep your livewire *currently* gets in a typical day. If it seems different every day, that's okay. If you haven't been tracking your little one's sleep, now is a good time to start.

WORKBOOK TO DO

Step #1: Refer to the Current Sleep Tracker in the Workbook (or use a sleep-tracking app or even just a sheet of paper). Start keeping track of your livewire's *current* sleep patterns for a few days.

Step #2: After you've gathered this information, use the New Daily Schedule Worksheet for your child's age to input the following information under the "Now" column. (It's okay to generalize. We know every day can be different.)

- How many naps are they getting per day (if applicable)?
- About how much time is there between wake-up and nap, between naps, and between the last nap and bedtime (i.e., what are their current awake windows)?
- What's their total nap / Quiet Time amount (approximately) for the day?
- What time is lights out at bedtime and what time are they actually asleep?
- How much total nighttime sleep are they getting?

Step #3: Use the following table to compare your livewire's current sleep to the targets for their age. Fill in the "Target" column on the worksheet accordingly.

SLEEP TARGETS BY AGE

Age	Awake window	No. of naps	Nap amount	Nighttime total
6–8 mos	2 hours	3	3½ hours	11 hours
9–10 mos	2–3 hours	2	3½ hours	11 hours
11–12 mos	3–4 hours	2	2½ hours	11 hours
13–17 mos	4–6 hours	2	2¼–2½ hours	11¼ hours
18–23 mos	5–6 hours	1	2¼ hours	11¼ hours
2 years	5–6 hours	1	2 hours	11 hours
3 years	6+ hours	1	1½ hours	10½ hours
4 years+	6+ hours	Nap or Quiet Time	45–60 minutes	11 hours

What do you notice? Is your livewire off by a lot? (Thirty minutes, give or take, isn't a huge deal. An hour or more likely means they are overtired.)

It's important to mention again that these are *targets*, not rules. They are just a starting point. We're going to shoot for these targets *at first* and then see where your livewire's sweet spots for sleep timing and amount really are. For the time being, let's see what happens when you work on getting them as close to these targets as you can.

I know you might be thinking, Ha! My child has never napped that much in their life!

Yes, it's possible that your livewire may do just fine on a little less sleep. Every child is different in terms of sleep needs—and this is *especially* true for livewires. However, I'm going to invite you, for the short-term, to give this a shot. If you really go for it and still find that your livewire doesn't hit the target, that's okay. Or you really try for a shorter wake window for a week, and they still fall asleep for a nap at the same time they always have.

It's important to see what happens if you give it a solid try to get them at least in the *neighborhood* of their target.

Kim and I have worked with a lot of parents who are convinced that their child needs far less sleep than is recommended simply because they can't get their livewire to sleep any longer than they are. When we start making a dent in the overtired / wired cycle by getting them enough well-timed naps, these same livewires often start napping longer and sleeping more at night. More sleep results in more sleep. Later in this chapter, we cover what to do if naps are just not in your control (like at daycare) or feel impossible because you have other children to attend to. Naps are hard, we know. Let's just try to move the needle if at all possible.

CRAFTING YOUR DAILY SCHEDULE

Even if you're not a "schedule" person (I wasn't, either), it's likely that your livewire *is*. Remember, livewires love a pattern, and they love predictability. If you can get your day organized so that there is a perceptible and consistent rhythm and there are predictable cues for naps (for example, there's always one right after lunch or after we have snack and read a book) and bedtime (we'll cover this in the next chapter), your livewire may settle in and start anticipating rest times. They still may not love it, but they'll know it's coming, and you can at least prevent those meltdowns that happen because your livewire is surprised that it's already naptime or bedtime. Give it a try to see if the benefits of a schedule outweigh any drawbacks to having a little more structure to the day. Your livewire will let you know if it's working or not.

Here are some sample schedules by age to give you an idea of how the day could look. These are intended to show you how naps and bedtime *could* be timed across a day. You will need to tweak and adjust based on your one-of-a-kind kiddo.

Example daytime schedules by age

Note: These are just examples. You can shift the times earlier or later based on when your family / child wakes for the day.

Six to Nine Months (Three Naps)

7 or 7:30 AM	Wake up for the day.
9 or 9:30 AM	Start nap 1: 1½ to 2 hours.
12:30 or 1 PM	Start nap 2: 1½ to 2 hours.
3 or 4 PM	Start nap 3: 45 minutes to 1 hour (all napping done by 5 PM or so).
6 or 6:30 PM	Start routine.
7 or 7:30 PM	Lights out.

Nine to Ten Months (Two Naps)

7 or 7:30 AM	Wake up for the day.
9 or 9:30 AM	Start nap 1: 1½ to 2 hours. (Once sleeping through the night, this nap can start three hours after wake-up instead of two, pushing nap #2's start time to 2 to 3 PM.)
1 or 2 PM	Start nap 2: 1½ to 2 hours (depending on the length of the first nap).
6 or 6:30 PM	Start routine.
7 or 7:30 PM	Lights out.

Eleven to Seventeen Months (Two Naps)

7 or 7:30 AM	Wake up for the day.
9 or 9:30 AM	Start nap 1: 1 to 1½ hours (can be three hours after wake-up once sleeping through the night).
1 or 2 PM	Start nap 2: 1 to 1½ hours (depending on length of first nap).
6 or 6:30 PM	Start routine.
7 or 7:30 PM	Lights out.

Eighteen Months and Up

7 or 7:30 AM	Wake up for the day.
12:30 or 1 PM	Start nap.
	Eighteen months to two years: 2¼ hours.
	Two years: 2 hours.
	Three years: 1½ hours.
	Four years and up: 45 minutes to 1 hour (nap or Quiet Time).
6 or 6:30 PM	Start routine.
7 or 8 PM	Lights out.

DEVELOPMENTAL CHANGES IN NAP AMOUNT AND TIMING

The number and length of naps children need changes across the first three or four years. These changes in daytime sleep structure typically happen somewhat naturally, as the brain develops and wake windows lengthen.

If a child is sleeping through the night, the three-to-two nap shift happens around nine months. The big caveat here is that, even though they are now taking only two naps, nine-month-olds still need *three-and-a-half hours* of daytime sleep. This transition only works if your livewire can take two good, long naps. If they can't, stick with shorter, more frequent naps until they get the hang of longer sleep. Often naps really improve once the child has learned to sleep at night.

The two-to-one nap shift happens at some point between fifteen and eighteen months (and really, it's most often closer to eighteen months). Kim has found that you will start seeing one or the other nap become more and more difficult to get (if they take a morning nap, for example, they won't take the afternoon one). Once you see this natural shift, you can start gradually moving either the morning nap later or the afternoon nap earlier, dropping whichever one seems to be harder to get, until you finally get to one midday (two or two-and-a-quarter-hour) nap.

> ## WORKBOOK TO DO
>
> Now, let's put it all together. Fill in the "New Schedule" section of the Daily Schedule Worksheet in the Workbook. What is your new rough schedule for the day? Look again at how much naptime you are going to need to shoot for, as well as the maximum window for your livewire's awake time.

TIPS FOR HITTING THOSE NAP TARGETS

Remember that these sleep targets don't have to be perfect—just better than they are now. We want to get your livewire at least a little closer to the daytime sleep amounts for their age. Here are some strategies to help you get there.

Regulate their morning wake-up time.

Try to have a limit on how late your child sleeps in the morning. This will give some consistency to your day and help set your child's inner body clock. A consistent start time for the day results in a more consistent bedtime, which has been shown to positively influence sleep patterns.[40] If your child is in daycare, the decision about when they should wake up may be made for you. But if wake-up time *is* up to you, consider waking your child by 7:30 or 8 AM at the latest so that the day's schedule stays on track.

If your child is sleeping in until 8 AM routinely and that works for your family, you can definitely get away with an 8 or 8:30 PM bedtime—but *only* if your child will sleep their full eleven hours. If they're waking at 6 AM, that later bedtime isn't going to work.

Watch the clock.

For the short-term, we want you to watch the clock so you can get them down before the end of their wake window. For example, if their wake window is two hours (refer back to the table on page 115), start observing them closely at about ninety minutes of awake time to see if they exhibit subtle tired signals that you may not have noticed before (spacing out, red eyebrows, etc.). The goal is to start the wind down for nap ahead of the end of their wake window—even if they appear to be going strong. *Do not wait.* See what happens. If the previous nap (or the previous night) was terrible, experiment with a window that's even shorter than the table says. With livewires, parents tend to go longer because they're waiting for their child to look tired. We're going to encourage you to experiment with always going *shorter* instead.

Have some transition / wind-down time ahead of the nap.

Livewires crank on all cylinders, and they don't do well with abrupt transitions. Having clear naptime cues (like a song, a chime, or dimmed lights starting a few minutes before) and then a short nap routine can really help them downshift and transition into rest mode. You don't want your livewire to feel blindsided when you suddenly walk them into their room for a nap. You want to give them a head start and clear cues. Daycares and preschools are great at this. They have repetitive routines and predictable signals for what's going to happen. If your child is in daycare or preschool and they nap well there, find out what the providers do before naptime and do exactly that.

TROUBLESHOOTING NAPS AND SCHEDULES

It's easy to *say* what wake windows and targets we're shooting for. Whether your livewire will follow those targets is another story. There are always outlier kiddos who want to carve their own way through their day. Here are some common nap quandaries and ways to navigate through them.

"What if I try all of these nap strategies and my child still won't nap very long (even if it's a contact nap)?"

Can I tell you how common this is? The idea behind knowing wake windows and trying for a nap sooner rather than later is to see if your livewire is

amenable to these adjustments. Some of them are and some of them aren't.
If naps are routinely really short, try shortening the next wake window(s) so
that you can possibly sneak in an extra one to get them closer to their nap
target. If *that* doesn't work, try taking them into a darker room and having
some chill time. At least they'll get a little sensory break. It's not as good
as a nap, but with persistent I'm-the-boss-of-me livewires, all you can do is
your best.

If we can get livewires to have better nights, sometimes naps get better
by themselves. But naps can still be super hard even after nighttime is good.
I had a client with a ten-month-old who didn't really sleep day *or* night.
The parents successfully coached the baby to sleep through the night and
then mom worked on naps hard for two solid weeks—but her livewire baby
would still only take one two-hour nap. Even after two weeks of effort,
that nap did not budge. Because nighttime was so good, we ended up just
accepting that this nap pattern worked for this particular baby.

We're mostly concerned with how short naps affect nighttime sleep.
We should *try* to improve naps, but once nighttime is handled, naps may
have to just be the way they are. We might have to accept that we have a
power-napper who gets all the rest they need in much less time than they're
supposed to.

"What happens on a really bad nap day?"

When there's the inevitable bad nap day where your livewire skips a nap, or
their last nap is so short that there is too much time left before bedtime, it
means that you can't just power through with your usual schedule.

Workaround #1: Emergency backup nap. If there is a surefire(ish)
method for getting your child to nap (car ride, stroller walk, lying with
them), *do that*, even if it's just for thirty minutes. If they don't sleep, at
least they're getting a little zone-out time.

Workaround #2: Earlier bedtime. Any time that naps are off kilter in
terms of timing or quantity, move bedtime earlier. This does not mean

that your livewire will wake up earlier. Just the opposite. By having an earlier bedtime, you are adding the missed naptime onto nighttime. You are also preventing even more overtired / wired bedtime behavior.

"What happens if daycare has a schedule that makes naps hard or impossible?"

Daycare can be a *really* challenging environment for livewires who need a lot of "just right" conditions to sleep. The noise and activity of a daycare setting can cause some livewires to have real trouble powering down. Plus, many daycares have policies or schedules that are challenging for children. Many facilities will move a one-year-old to a room with only one nap. Because the transition from two naps to one happens closer to eighteen months, this can result in an overtired kiddo at pickup. Some daycares have a 1 to 3 PM naptime, and that can be late for little ones who are early risers. Some daycares won't wake a sleeping child or don't have ways to make the room quieter or darker. There are a lot of ways that daycare can be difficult for a child who's not a super good sleeper, meaning that parents are picking up an overtired child at the end of a busy day.

While you may not have a ton of options if your livewire struggles to nap at daycare (except to hope they adjust over time), here are a few things you can try.

Talk to your provider about what's possible in terms of adjustments to either the setting or schedule. See if you can negotiate the quietest, darkest spot for your livewire and if you can bring in a white noise gadget. Kim has worked with some livewires whose parents had to find a smaller daycare setting that was more conducive to sleep. If your baby just can't sleep for their morning nap because toddlers are loudly playing nearby, some daycares will be willing to put them down at the other end of the open room. Can your provider rock your baby to sleep, or back to sleep if they only nap briefly? See if there are strategies they can offer you.

Get daily information / logs from your provider on your child's nap timing and length. If you know when and how much they napped during the day, you can respond accordingly—getting them a little nap in the car on the way home and/or moving bedtime earlier if they're coming home short on daytime sleep.

"What do I do about naps when they wake too early for the day (before 6 AM)?"

One of the big problems with a predawn wake-up (besides it being god-awful early) is what to do about naps. If your little one wakes at 5 AM, it's going to be hard to make it to their usual bedtime with just their usual amount of naptime, and without a bigger-than-desired wake window somewhere in there. You also don't necessarily want them going to bed at 5 PM because that can result in an early bedtime / early wake-up cycle.

Early wake-ups are often a result of overtiredness and/or not having solid sleep skills. One part of resolving early rising is making sure they're not overtired. Here are two options for how to do that, with examples based on a nine-month-old:

Option #1: Give an extra nap.

5 AM	Wake up for the day (oof).
6:30 AM	Start extra nap (45 minutes or less).
(Or as soon as they look sleepy.)	
9:30 AM	Start nap 1 (as usual, 90 minutes to 2 hours).
1:30 PM	Start nap 2 (as usual, 90 minutes to 2 hours).
7 PM	Lights out.

In this example, you are giving them an extra nap (something I like to call a nap snack) that you can consider a continuation of nighttime sleep. Then, they'll be on their regular nap schedule, with two-hour wake windows. You could also try this nap snack at the end of the day instead if that works better for your livewire. In either case, this extra daytime sleep helps your child make it to a reasonable bedtime.

Important note: This is only a *temporary* strategy to disrupt early rising while still preserving a relatively normal bedtime. Once that wake-up returns to its usual time, you should go back to your regular daytime nap schedule. Remember that early rising is stubborn. It can take a week or more to resolve. (See chapter twelve for more about how to assess and address early rising.)

Option #2: Have an earlier (but not *too* much earlier) bedtime.

5 AM	Wake up for the day.
8 AM	Start nap 1 (90 minutes to 2 hours).
12 PM	Start nap 2 (90 minutes to 2 hours).
6 PM	Lights out.

Here, you put your child down for just the two naps that they usually have, but much earlier because of the early wake-up. In this option, bedtime is backed up by an hour or more to account for lost sleep from the night before and to prevent your child from being up for five or more hours straight. You will have to experiment with that wake window before bed. Often, this window can be a little longer. Test out whether a longer window helps bedtime without making them over-tired / wired.

It's important to emphasize that we don't want you getting stuck here in this early bedtime pattern. As you move forward, you'll want to start pushing that first nap a little later while continuing to work on keeping the nap tank full.

There's no right or wrong here. Test to see which one of these options works better for your livewire. If you decide on option 2 (no extra nap / earlier bedtime) and they're a mess in the afternoon, or those naps were harder to get or shorter than their target, you will know that the wake window from 5 AM to their earlier nap at 8 AM was just too long, and you'll need to go with option 1 (offering the extra nap).

After addressing potential overtiredness, the next important part of tackling early rising is going to be working on those go-to-sleep skills, which we will cover in chapter nine. Once they master those sleep skills and their daytime nap timing and amount are on point, early rising should resolve . . . eventually. You may have to hang in there a bit (a week or two) before it budges.

"What if I have more than one child?"

Organizing a good nap schedule when there are siblings to contend with is not always easy (or even possible). The baby needs to nap, but you have to pick up the older child at preschool. The older child needs to nap, but you have a newborn and can't go lie with them for an hour. This is just a reality. Our message here is this: You have to do what you have to do. You may need to hand the newborn off or see if they will hang out in a safe space so you can lie down with your toddler or take them both for a car ride. Get creative and try to hit the nap targets, but know you may have to just live with a schedule that's not ideal.

"What if we really want to have dinner together or we don't get home until six or seven?"

This is so understandable. Bedtime is supposed to be 7 PM (and the bedtime routine starts even earlier), but your child gets picked up from daycare at 5:30 or 6 PM, or one parent doesn't get home until then, and there's barely time for dinner, much less playtime. You will have to weigh the positives and negatives of keeping them up later. Yes, you get some precious time with your child in the evenings. But young children who need to be up early to be at school or childcare also need an early bedtime. Pushing it later can mean a cranky-pants child at dinnertime, more bedtime struggles, and more night waking. Plus, while making bedtime a priority can mean sacrificing some evening (after work) family time, it won't be forever. And you may find that the cost of less time in the evening buys you an easier bedtime and a better night (not a bad trade-off).

The right bedtime has to account for what time everyone needs to be up in the morning. If you all have to be up by 7:30 AM to be out of the house by 8 AM, your child needs to be asleep by 7:30 PM or so to get the recommended eleven hours (not including wake-ups or time for feeds). If your child doesn't have to get up early for school or daycare *and* they'll sleep until 8 AM, a slightly later bedtime may work for your family. As long as your child is sleeping well, it doesn't really matter what time bedtime is. Just make sure your little one is getting the amount of nighttime sleep that they need.

ONWARD WE GO . . .

Once you have a good daytime nap schedule and a good early bedtime that keeps your child from getting the dreaded second wind, it's time to work on setting up a successful bedtime routine. With livewires, preparation is everything. Ready?

OUR TRIP CHECKLIST

- ☑ You know you are on a different path.
- ☑ You understand your livewire's temperament strengths and challenges.
- ☑ You understand the link between temperament and sleep issues.
- ☑ Your child is ready:
  - ☑ Over six months
  - ☑ No upcoming disruptions
  - ☑ No physiological issues that affect sleep
- ☑ You are ready (or as ready as you can be).
- ☑ You understand the Big Four sources of sleep issues.

- ☑ **Big Strategy #1: You know how to avoid that second wind.**
- ☐ Big Strategy #2: You have a solid, consistent bedtime routine.
- ☐ Big Strategy #3 and #4: You know how to change the go-to-sleep and back-to-sleep patterns and are prepared to be more consistent than you've ever been before.
- ☐ You know how to track progress.
- ☐ You know how to diagnose and fix any problems that arise.
- ☐ BETTER SLEEP!

CHAPTER 8

Big Strategy #2: Have an Effective Lead-Up to Lights Out

The Magic of a Solid Bedtime Routine

If you are finding yourself dreading the dumpster fire that is bedtime, you are not alone. Ending the day with meltdowns (theirs and/or yours) or feeling trapped and resentful sitting in the dark for an hour or more waiting for your livewire to finally go the heck to sleep is not how we want things to be. The key to a less stressful bedtime is careful preparation. Investing time in planning can reduce the struggles and shenanigans and can give your livewire some predictable cues about what is going to happen so they're not caught off guard. Trust me, with livewires, preparation is *everything*.

All day, livewires are busy, their brain humming with the massive amount of learning and experiencing they are doing. They simply can't stop their exciting day on a dime to brush their teeth, read a book, and go to sleep. Livewires require buckets of transition time. The older the livewire, the more time (and preparation on your part) they need to be mentally and physically ready for sleep.

In this chapter, we'll give you a whole menu of possible strategies to help you craft a predictable and sustainable plan that starts way before bedtime.

You can pick and choose among these strategies based on what will work best for your unique child at their particular stage of development. Not all the strategies will work for every livewire. Use what you know about which actions rev them up (talking, picture books, etc.) and which help them calm down (listening to recorded stories, etc.) to craft your plan. Also, even though we've roughly grouped some of the strategies by age, feel free to go by what your child is able to do and use the strategies you think will work.

HOW DEVELOPMENT IMPACTS WHAT YOU NEED TO DO AT BEDTIME

Our second big strategy, having an effective lead-up to lights out, is about laying the groundwork for shifting their sleep patterns by setting them (and you) up for success. We want to remove as many obstacles as we can. First, it's important to understand the ways that development can impact how much prep you need to do for bedtime.

Infants and toddlers. Babies and toddlers, as a rule, need and like cues and predictable routines. For perceptive, easily thrown livewires, these can be even more important. Livewires love a predictable pattern. If we can establish one and stick with it, they seem to appreciate the heads-up about what's going to happen.

At these early ages, routines and patterns can be easy and not terribly involved. They just need to be consistent night to night. We're going to set you up with a routine that makes sense so that you can ease into bedtime without a lot of drama.

Two-year-olds. Developmentally, the second birthday comes with a big cognitive milestone that can directly impact bedtime and nighttime. The reason *no* is such a popular word at this age is that they are just now discovering that they can have different thoughts than you have . . . and *no* is their way of expressing that. Suddenly, they *don't* want to lie down and go to sleep. They *don't* want their lovey. They use all their considerable abilities to try to get you to stay with them, rock them, etc., and with that active, creative, sharp livewire brain behind them, they really know what they're doing.

None of this needs to stop your work on sleep. In fact, having a predictable routine with limited options is going to be helpful for this. Being "separate" is exciting for a toddler, but also a little daunting. Consistent routines and limits are good for them because they let your child know that you are always there to steer the ship.

Three-year-olds (and up). I find that parents are often surprised at the level of sleep challenges they can have with three-year-olds. Three is an incredibly common moment for sleep problems to rear their heads. Why? I'm just going to say it: *Three-year-olds are drunk with power.* And the power trip may not end any time soon. At this stage, livewires are *on fire* with their own potential and ability. Not only can they have their own thoughts, they can also use their considerable verbal and cognitive skills to *make what they think about happen.* They can look at a situation and think, *How can I change this to something I like better?*

Most of the time, it's an awesome thing to witness. At bedtime, however? Not so much. Especially when they are no longer corralled in a crib. Bedtime can easily become a circus full of drawn-out struggle, negotiation, and frustration (meltdowns, yelling, begging, pleading). Seven books? Four songs? Holding their parent's hair while they fall asleep? Drink of water? Coming out of their room a zillion times? A bespoke story about their day? Parents can tie themselves into crazy knots just to get their livewires ready to go the heck to sleep. Don't worry if this is you. It's par for the course with livewires.

With older livewires (three and up, but some two-and-a-half-year-olds, too), you will need even *more* preparation to stay ahead of the shenanigan parade. We're going to suggest a few additional wind-down strategies, then we're going to lock down how many options they have during the routine. We're going to give them plenty of heads-up and rehearsal for anything that's going to be changing. Our main goal is to prevent any surprises from happening at bedtime and you, the parent, from having to make any decisions in the moment or on the fly. When you are wiped out, you know how hard it can be to say no to a random request. Suddenly, you're reading eight books, offering snacks, and performing an interpretive dance at bedtime, wondering how you got here. Planning and preparation will be your friend.

CRAFTING YOUR LEAD-UP TO LIGHTS OUT

> ### WORKBOOK TO DO
>
> For these next sections, you are going to want to have the Bedtime Routine Worksheet downloaded or have a notebook handy to make notes as you go. This chapter is going to give you *lots* of options, and you really can pick and choose which strategies you think will work for you and your livewire. We're going to walk through all the preliminary planning you'll need to do to set yourself up for success.

STEP #1: DECIDE WHERE SLEEP IS GOING TO HAPPEN

Where is your child sleeping now? Is that working for you? Do you need to make a change? If so, now can be a great time to make a move: new space, new plan. There are lots of ways for everyone to get good sleep, and as long as you know the upsides and potential downsides of each choice, you can make whatever decision you want for yourself and your family. The key question is this: Is everyone sleeping well?

Here are some things to consider, especially if where you want them to sleep is different from where they're sleeping now.

Moving to a crib in their own room (six months and up)

While there are no hard-and-fast rules for having a baby sleep in their own room after six months, I can tell you after working with many sensitive parents of sensitive kiddos that having *everyone* in the same room is a mixed bag. On the one hand, it feels easier to have them close by when you're getting up a lot. However, remember that livewires have very thin sensory barriers. Even mundane sounds that happen at night—someone sneezing or snoring, someone rustling the sheets as they turn over—can cause an engaged livewire to wake and think, *Oh, right! Mom and Dad are right there!* Sometimes, getting a livewire in their own space can be super helpful.

If you're moving your livewire from a crib or bassinet in your room (or even from co-sleeping) to a crib in their own room, give them some day-time playtime in the new space once it's set up—before you start working on sleep—so that they develop positive associations with it. You may want to have a mattress in there for yourself for the first few nights of coaching, just as a transition and to be able to get to them quickly. For folks who have been co-sleeping, you could co-sleep on a mattress with them for a few days before transitioning them to the crib. Just don't get stuck sleeping in their room for much longer than that. Make sure you're back in your own room in less than a week.

Continuing to co-sleep (all ages)

This choice is totally okay as long as the space is safe (yada, yada . . . you know the drill) and *everyone* sleeps well. If you're co-sleeping and both parents and child can sleep, that's awesome. Co-sleeping works great . . . until it doesn't. Remember, sensitive livewires can be light sleepers, and the movement and sound of a shared sleep surface can cause them to wake. Add to this a sensitive parent who wakes at every sound the *baby* makes, and you have a recipe for bad sleep all around. It's important to decide where every-one sleeps best. If you had your heart set on co-sleeping but you or your baby (or both of you) aren't sleeping well, you may need to pivot. There may be ways to split the difference (for example, only co-sleep after 5 AM) that we will cover in chapter ten.

I co-slept with both of my children. It worked great with my daughter, and she moved easily to her own space at two-and-a-half once my son came along. My son and I, however, were both extremely light sleepers. He was waking every forty-five minutes until well over a year old. I liked co-sleeping, but for the two of us, it was not working. In retrospect, I think both of us would have slept much better in separate spaces (or even just on separate surfaces). We just didn't know how to make that happen at the time.

Infants. Even if co-sleeping is working for you and you want to continue, we're going to suggest that you *consider* coaching your baby to sleep in a crib or pack and play, at least for bedtime and the first part of the night until you go to bed. Then you can co-sleep the rest of the night. It's really not safe to have infants sleep alone on a big bed, especially once they're mobile. Another perk? If they are sleeping in a contained space, *you* don't have to go to bed when the baby does. You might just get a few hours of being a grown-up before going to bed. (Can I tell you how many parents I've worked with who have not had an evening with their partner in who knows how long?) Working on at least a few crib skills (specifics in chapter ten) will also give your live-wire some skills in case you ever—I don't know—get a babysitter and go out for an evening.

Toddlers and up. Co-sleeping is a great strategy if everyone sleeps well. We will talk about how to modify sleep coaching if there's still a lot of night nursing or bottles happening. It *is* possible to both co-sleep and work to get better sleep for everyone.

Moving to a floor bed or toddler bed (children under three)

Very often, the move to a floor bed in younger children is a response to an agile little livewire who has (or totally could) take a header out of the crib. If there is literally no way to safely keep your child in the crib, the floor bed decision has been made for you. On the other hand, parents sometimes choose a floor bed thinking it will improve their livewire's problematic sleep, hoping that the extra space may help. Or they're convinced that their little one hates the crib. Or maybe they've read about or are attending a Montessori daycare and are consciously choosing a floor bed as part of this philosophy. Regardless of the reason, a child under three on a floor bed presents some challenges that accompany all that extra freedom. It's definitely an option—just make sure you are aware of (and plan for) the possible hurdles.

With floor beds, it's important to think beyond right now. A floor bed for a baby who isn't yet crawling might work, but what happens when they are more mobile? Without the walls of a crib, your wily, whip-smart live-wire will no longer be safely contained. It's going to be important to con-sider the room (what can be climbed, what can be tossed around / emptied) and how you might keep them in there at night without this becoming your new bedroom.

A smart toddler in a bed is going to up the rodeo quotient by a lot. Before three, children may *know*, cognitively, that you want them to stay in bed, but they aren't yet able to use that knowledge to keep themselves there. They don't yet have the impulse control to stay in their bed or their room. Without a crib keeping them contained, you can be in for a daunting amount of walking them back to their bed over and over.

If you have a world-class climber / budding Olympic athlete, we sug-gest seeing if you can prevent the climbing. Keeping a younger child in the crib is going to be easier (believe it or not) than dealing with the can of worms that freedom is going to open. Here are a few strategies to keep them corralled for a little longer:

- Lower the mattress all the way to the floor.
- If that doesn't work or isn't possible, there are pajamas with a band sewn between the legs that prevent little Houdinis from raising a leg enough to climb. (You can also try sleep sacks that do some-thing similar.)
- Securely install a safe crib tent.

If these options don't work and you are really worried for their safety, you may have no choice but to move them to a floor mattress or toddler bed and accept that staying in bed may not be in their wheelhouse for a while. Really childproof the room (anchor dressers, remove a lot of toys, etc.).

A baby gate or a door strap (a gadget that only allows the door to open a smidge) will help keep your little one from wandering the house at night.

Don't get us wrong, beds for children under three *can* work, but you may need to lower your expectations a little for your work on sleep skills. In the absence of some sort of containment, sleep coaching can take longer and there may be pieces of the sleep picture that don't totally fall into place until they developmentally mature a little more. All that said, some kiddos really do well with it, and as long as you know the additional challenges it can present for both sleep coaching and safety, you'll go into it prepared. (Still, maybe don't give away the crib just yet. You can always pull it back out if the floor bed is a bust.)

Moving to a big kid bed (three years and up)

If sleeping in a big kid bed is going to be new to your child, there are a few steps you can take to make this transition easier. Big kid beds don't have the same sense of containment a crib does, and some livewires can feel a little lost in all that open space. If this is the case for yours, you may want to consider a canopy or tent for the bed so that it feels a little more enclosed. Body pillows can make great bolsters if your livewire likes to feel cozy. Let them pick out sheets and pillowcases to make the space their own. Most importantly, prepare them ahead of time with a conversation and maybe even some rehearsal during the day. Picture books about big kid beds can also reinforce how to navigate this new experience. (Don't worry, we're going to say a lot more about this below when we talk about the bedtime routine.)

You'll also have some decisions to make:

Do you expect them to sleep in their own room / bed all night, or just part of the night? Before you start, it's important to decide whether they need to stay in their own bed all night or not. Are you going to insist that their room is the only place they sleep? Is there ever a situation when it's okay for them to co-sleep? Or do you want to establish a floor bed in your room where they can go in the middle of the night?

Any of these options are fine. However, for the options that allow your child to come into your room, it's important to decide when and how all of that will happen.

Is there a set a time after which it's okay for them to come into your room? You might decide that you want your livewire in their room until, say, 3 AM, when they most often wake. That's a fine line to draw. (You really can pick any time that makes sense to you. The key is that they're spending *some* of the night in their own space. You can work on stretching that time as you move forward.) You'll need to have a wake-up clock that turns on or changes color to let them know when it's okay to come *quietly* into your room.

Do you have requirements for how and where they can sleep in your room? If it's okay for them to come into your room in the middle of the night, they should be in charge of being as quiet as they possibly can. There's no need for them to wake you. Is it okay to climb in bed with you? If not, create a space on the floor that's got fun sheets and a pillow.

Moving in with a sibling

If you are thinking of moving your child in with an older sibling, it usually doesn't work to sleep coach with the sibling in the room. We suggest *temporarily* moving the sibling out and having them sleep somewhere else. (If that place is on the floor of your room, be sure the sibling understands this is *temporary*, so you don't accidentally create a new problem.) Coach your child in the new space, and then, once they're sleeping well, move the sibling back in.

STEP #2: MAKE SURE THE SLEEP LOCATION IS LIVEWIRE FRIENDLY

An active, alert brain and low sensory threshold mean that it's difficult (if not impossible) for livewires to tune anything out. Once you decide where they will be sleeping at night, that sleep environment needs to be set up in a way that encourages winding down and disconnecting from the excitement of the waking world. This is about more than cute bedding or pictures of clouds. Their sleep spaces need to take their unique sensory needs and sensitivities into account. In crafting both their sleep space and bedtime routines, you will need to think carefully about what kinds of sensory input cause them to wake up, what annoys them, what helps them relax, etc.

Here are a few things to think about:

Is the room too interesting? We don't want anything in the sleep environment that will distract your visually alert livewire from the business of powering down. If you find that instead of going to sleep, they force their eyes open to look at decorations on the walls, it may be time to make the room a little more, well, *boring*. You may need to reduce the number of toys or books in the room. When in doubt, less is more. If you notice anything grabbing their attention, it's got to go for now. You can potentially reintroduce decorations or toys once sleep is handled.

How are the light levels? How bright is the room? Some children need total darkness to fall asleep. Blackout curtains or shades, or those new privacy bed tents, can give little ones a little darkness and even a cozy feeling of containment. Parents often wonder about night-lights. Use them? Don't use them? For a while, there was some worrisome research circulating about the effect of artificial light on children's sleep and vision.[41] However, that research has largely been refuted.[42] You just have to ask yourself: Does a little light help or hurt your livewire's ability to fall asleep? This is another area where you can just test it out. Light or no light? Brighter or dimmer? Different colors? Maybe the light needs to be somewhere else in the room. Observe your livewire, and see what works (or doesn't).

What about white noise? White noise is almost a necessity for helping livewires fall asleep (not always, but often). While there have been some scary posts on social media about the effect of white noise on children's hearing and language development, you should know that this research was focused on the effect of noise pollution (constant loud noise).[43]

Research on sound levels produced by white noise devices suggests that devices be kept several feet away from the crib / bed, and the volume used be less than fifty decibels (there are apps that will help you measure this).[44] If you can get away with turning the white noise off at some point in the night, that's great (but if not, don't worry about it). Experiment to see whether white noise works for your child and then try to use the lowest level you can get away with.

For livewires not in a crib: Childproofing is a must. If your livewire is mobile and not contained in a crib, you will need to childproof the heck out of the room by removing or securing things that can fall or be pulled down or slammed shut on small fingers. You may also need to install a baby gate or door strap to prevent them from roaming the house at night.

STEP #3: HELP THEM TRANSITION INTO BEDTIME WITH A PRE-ROUTINE ROUTINE

Mellower kiddos may need very little cuing that it's time to put toys away and start the bedtime routine. They may grumble, but they will get moving within a reasonable timeframe. Livewires, as a rule, need *tons* of warning and transition time to move from fun time / awake time to boring old sleep time. Before the routine even starts, livewires often need a transition *into* the transition. Signaling ahead of time that the pace is about to slow down can help you avoid surprising them with *"Okay, it's time for bed!"* and then—*kaboom!*—the meltdown that ensues because they didn't see it coming. Let's talk about a few clear steps you can add before you're ready to start the bedtime routine.

A WORD ABOUT SCREEN TIME BEFORE BED

It's tempting to use a video or a few minutes of a favorite show as a surefire way to help little livewires downshift. Unfortunately, research has clearly shown that the light that gets emitted from screens, including phones and tablets, disrupts the evening release of melatonin, and believe me, you are going to want every microgram of melatonin on your side. The research is pretty clear on the effect of blue light and screen time on kids' sleep.[45] If you *really* need a quick dose of a video, try to use the function on phones and computers that blocks blue light. And do your best to turn off screens about an hour before lights out. (Also, no TVs in children's rooms. Research has shown that a TV in a bedroom is a direct cause of much poorer sleep.)[46]

Pre-routine routines for babies and toddlers

Even preverbal little ones need some signaling that bedtime is coming so they can navigate the transition. Remember, many livewires don't cope well with sudden shifts between activities. About a half hour before you're ready to *start* the bedtime routine, gradually start lowering the lights, turn off the TV, and maybe have a song or other signal that the bedtime routine is about to start. For toddlers who are old enough to understand, a toy cleanup routine can be a signal that playing time is done. Whatever you choose, do it in the same sequence every night so that these actions clue your child in that bedtime is coming.

Pre-routine routines for three(ish) years and up

Remember that older toddlers and preschoolers are going to need *much more* prep on your part before bedtime. This is part shenanigan prevention and part consistency insurance. Having a fun activity that always happens *before* the routine starts is a great way to prep them for the nighttime transition. They won't even notice that these are strategies to get them ready for bedtime. It's like sneaking veggies into their dessert.

Here are two activities that are easy to do and can be *magic*.

Special Time

Special Time is an incredibly easy research-based activity with massive payoffs.[47] Special Time involves fifteen to twenty minutes (not ten—fifteen to twenty) of your 100 percent undivided attention every night before the bedtime routine where the child gets to be The Boss. They tell *you* what they want to play and what they want you to be, say, and do. For this period of time, they are in charge (within reason). This is their time with you or your partner. Special Time can be a great way to transition from the after-dinner bustle into getting ready for bed. I often suggest doing Special Time in their room so that you're already in the chute for the bedtime routine.

For livewires with active brains and who have a lot of opinions about how bedtime should go, Special Time gives them an opportunity to get some of that out of their system by giving them a little dose of agency and power *before* the bedtime routine starts. For livewires who have a new younger sibling, Special Time may be even more important. It gives them some one-on-one time with parents who may otherwise be occupied with a new baby, so that they don't have to try to work for that attention *during* the routine. But even if you think that your livewire gets a ton of attention during the day (and we're sure they do), Special Time still works. It's a simple, doable few minutes that can have huge payoffs at bedtime (and beyond).

What your livewire chooses to do during Special Time can sometimes give you a little window into what they're thinking about, too. Children communicate via play, so pay attention to what they are saying and doing during this time. You may get to learn a little about what's going on in that busy brain.

Heavy work

If you have a kiddo who is jumping and running and powering up just as it's time to turn out the lights, this activity is for you. Heavy work isn't actually *work*. It comes from the field of occupational therapy and includes fun activities that can help active livewires use their body in ways that ultimately help them slow down. Heavy work provides big input via activities that engage the big muscles and joints of the body. Activities like pushing, pulling, jumping, or crashing help them wind down, believe it or not, so that they're not bouncing off the walls like crazy people once it's time to get into bed. I know. It seems totally counterintuitive. *"Aren't we supposed to avoid roughhousing before bed?"* Yes, *usually*, but some livewires need that big input to calm down. Remember when you had to vigorously bounce them on a yoga ball before sleep as a baby? Being bounced, as opposed to gently rocked or swayed, is big input. This is essentially the same strategy.

Activities to try:

- Race down a hallway . . .
  - pushing a laundry basket full of books.
  - carrying a water jug.
  - walking like a spider.
- Do wheelbarrow walking (where you hold their feet and they walk on their hands).
- Make a pile of pillows or couch cushions and crash them into it.
- Play tug-of-war with a towel.
- Swing (in an actual playground swing, in an indoor fabric one, or even from an indoor pull-up bar).
- Swing them in a blanket if they're small enough.
- Jump for a few minutes on an indoor trampoline.
- Play with clay or Play-Doh.
- Blow bubbles.
- Drink a thick liquid (smoothie, applesauce) through a straw.

All these activities stimulate the big muscles and joints so that the child can physically downshift . . . and they're fun, so it's an easy segue into the routine.

STEP #4: CRAFT AN EFFECTIVE (AND MANAGEABLE) BEDTIME ROUTINE

A solid routine is important for laying the groundwork for sleep coaching all children. As they grow in cognitive ability as they age, the routine becomes even more important.

In this section, we've tried to group strategies by age as best we can, but as you read through this section, feel free to pick and choose what you think your unique kiddo might respond to. Just because it says it's for three-year-olds doesn't mean it won't work for your ahead-of-the-curve two-and-a-half-year-old.

In an effective lead-up to lights out, we want each step to help your child slow down and disconnect from the day so that falling asleep is easier. The main questions I want you to ask of each activity as you craft your routine are: Does this help? Does it make my livewire calm down a little, or is it making my job ten times more difficult?

You may have already found out the hard way that some bedtime routine staples don't work with livewires. Just because these are considered givens for a solid bedtime routine doesn't mean you have to include them—*especially* if they make things harder for you.

Baths. This may shock you, but baths aren't always calming for livewires and don't always make them sleepy. Water is a sensory experience that can do the opposite of what you are hoping for. I had a client with two little boys, and when I asked if the bath calmed them down, Mom said, "Good grief, no. They run around the house like maniacs after the bath." If it's party time after a bath, *don't do it at bedtime*. It may feel totally backward, but bath time may have to happen during the day. If you feel like it's necessary, you can just do a quick wipe down at bedtime.

Books and stories. Here's another shocker. For very visual and/or verbal livewires, stories with pictures can light up their brain instead of making them drowsy. Even for babies, the visual input can cause them to *engage*. If a picture book gets them mentally activated, you may need to save those for daytime.

Look at what kinds of books do and don't work. You may find that there are *types* of books that can be calming. Kim's livewire really liked books with intricate pictures that she could think about in bed. For other livewires, though, too much detail gets their brain churning with questions or ideas. You could potentially choose books that are more muted or have fewer pictures, or you could do something nonvisual like listening to music.

Bedtime routines for babies and toddlers up to three(ish) years

A good bedtime routine at this age doesn't have to be complicated or long—it just has to be consistent and *focused on helping your livewire slow down*. Then, after a little pre-routine downshifting, you can move toward the bedtime routine. At these early ages, we just want the last few steps to be the same. Besides the usual diaper change, book, song, etc., here are some sensory strategies that can help sensitive, alert little ones calm down by giving some pressure or compression to their bodies. This kind of input can help on-the-go livewires start to relax.

Additional strategies for babies and toddlers include:

Squeezy massages. Most massages for young ones use light, stroking motions. That *can* work for some livewires, but if yours is a sensory seeker and likes big input, stroking massages can be annoying for them. Instead, try a squeezy massage that gently but firmly compresses the joints and big muscles.

Blanket or towel burritos. Similarly, you can briefly wrap them tightly in a towel or blanket and do a gentle full-body squeeze, giving gentle compression to their whole body.

Gentle swinging. Some OTs suggest putting a child in a blanket, holding the ends, and gently swinging them back and forth. The compression plus the swinging motion is an effective, calming combo.

Additional strategies for two(ish) years and up include:

Bedtime yoga or stretching. There are a variety of books, videos, and recordings aimed at young children that teach simple, easy bedtime yoga poses and stretches that can encourage physical and mental downshifting.

Mindfulness / deep breathing. By about two, you can start teaching some basic techniques that slow your child's brain down by focusing on their breath and their body. There are great recordings and books that teach children how to breathe deeply and relax their bodies. An active, busy brain is going to hang around for the long-term. Giving livewires practical tools for slowing down, focusing on their breathing, and calming their body will have long-term benefits. Deep breathing can help at moments of big feelings (theirs *and* yours). We all can benefit from a few more deep breaths.

A BIG, MAJOR SLEEP ROUTINE CAVEAT: THE LAST STEP OF THE ROUTINE CAN'T BE A FEED

This goes for babies, of course, but also toddlers who may still have milk before bed. It's going to be critical to unhook feeding (or milk) from sleep for two reasons:

1. We don't want your child going into bed drowsier than you think (and milk is like a little sleeping pill for kiddos).
2. We want a little distance between feeding and sleep so that they understand going to sleep as a separate task.

This means that you need to put at least *one or two steps* between having milk and going into the crib. It's important to note that for children with teeth, dentists want those teeth to be brushed after milk because milk sugars can really increase the risk of early cavities.[48] We also don't want your livewire to be falling asleep with a bottle in their hands. It just becomes a major part of their go-to-sleep pattern.

Do the feed, *then* put on the sleep sack, read a book, etc., and *then* put them into the crib.

Here's what a potential routine could look like:

- Bath (or wipe down, if a bath is too stimulating)
- Squeezy massage, burrito roll, and/or swinging
- Diaper change, pajamas / sleep sack
- Feed / milk (nursing or bottle)
- Brush teeth (for toddlers)
- Story or song / music
- Say good night to the room
- White noise on / lights out
- Into bed

Remember, your routine doesn't have to be super long, just really, really, *really* consistent.

Bedtime routines for three(ish) years and up

At this age, preparation is everything. The more forethought you can put into bedtime, the better. Here's why: Smart, persistent livewires like to poke every rule, and they can become so frustrated when it doesn't go their way. With livewires three(ish) years and up, we're going to give lots of warning for how things are going to go, we're going to have an insane degree of predictability, and we're going to really lock down the opportunities for negotiation with a set-in-stone routine.

Before we get into the nitty-gritty of building the actual routine, how-ever, you need to know what type of bedtime challenge (or challenges) you need to address. There can be a host of additional bedtime obstacles at this age—especially with livewires, who use every bit of their mental skill to delay going to sleep. We're going to get you well-prepared for the curveballs they are going to lob your way. Knowing where the traps are is the first step toward being able to detour around them.

The Negotiator

This smart, perceptive, verbal livewire has the smarts and perceptiveness to poke every single limit you have. If you've ever said, "Okay, *just for tonight*," I'm sure you found out that that limit was now toast. *"If it was okay for last night, why not tonight?"* On the fly, you have no good answer for that, and now whatever you said yes to "just for tonight" is the new normal. Flexi-bility sends the message that limits are negotiable or potentially open for debate. Negotiator livewires will seize this opportunity. They will dig in their heels for what they want or at least what they think they can make happen. Your momentary fatigue-fueled wobble has now opened the door to a world of possibilities for your smart kiddo.

When you are this tired, who can blame you? It's easy (and totally com-mon) for parents to get so worn down that they resort to the path of least resistance and start bending the rules just because they can't take the fight that will follow. The problem with this is that you inadvertently end up giv-ing your dynamo way too much power. I've seen it happen a lot, and while I totally understand it (and lived it myself), this imbalance of power becomes a monkey wrench in the go-to-sleep process. Your livewire will continue to push harder and for longer because they believe it could potentially work.

With force-of-nature livewires who are kind of running the show, you also can't give them all the power during the day and then expect it to go well when you try to reclaim the driver's seat at bedtime. If you feel like you're really struggling to rein in your livewire day and night, get some professional input and support. This work can't just happen at bedtime.

Solutions

Front-load the requests. We are going to talk in the next section about how to create a Bedtime Chart. This chart is *not* a sticker chart (those don't really work for livewires anyway). It's a kind of contract between you and your child for what will (and won't) happen at bedtime. We're going to have you work with your livewire to craft a list of everything that will be part of their routine. Most importantly, you are going to be able to front-load the types of requests (another bathroom trip, drink of water, different lovey) that can be used to prolong the routine. You're going to craft the chart so that requests are agreed upon, planned, and happen *before* the lights go out.

The Bedtime Pass. This is a research-based strategy for those bedtime jack-in-the-boxes who just *will not* stay in bed and keep coming out for a million different reasons.[49] Make an actual piece of paper that has "Bedtime Pass" written on it (feel free to make it fancier than that if you want). It can be used for *one* request after the lights go out. After that, no more. If they don't use the pass, make sure you make a big deal about it. You may even consider giving some kind of reward (fun event / treat) when they hold on to it more than once in a week. It sounds way too simple and easy, I know, but there's research that shows that it works. The idea is that if a child knows they *can* use it (if they know it's an option), that may be all they need.

Be the decider. Negotiator livewires need solid, sustainable guidelines that are *immovable*. Once you decide on the routine, don't let it wobble even a little. If there's ever a moment when you must negotiate, *you* have to be the ultimate decision-maker. If you say, "I'll come back in ten minutes," and your livewire says, "Three minutes," you have to come back with either your original ten (the best choice) or another amount that's more than what they wanted. If they say three and you say, "Okay," the power dynamic is lopsided. Livewires need to know that you will be strong with the limits you set. This helps them because they don't have to worry that rules or events will shift easily. *Be the decider.*

Try sleep visualization stories. These are recorded guided visualizations for sleep disguised as stories about castles, or fairies, or dinosaurs. (They're available online and on a wide variety of apps.) These are great for livewires because the stories force them to listen and use their imagination in the service of relaxation. They can focus their attention on the story instead of all the thoughts of the day. Listening to a story is also great for very visual / verbal livewires for whom illustrated storybooks are like brain catnip.

The Talker

Oh, boy. This verbal, engaged livewire just wants to keep the conversation going. Lots of questions, lots of ideas, lots of thoughts about the day. This is awesome—but not at bedtime. Their uber active mind ramps up in response to thoughts, images, or ideas . . . all of which appear to come tumbling out just as the lights are going down. Their active brain is never going to stop being active, so giving them tools for learning how to drive it is going to have lifelong benefits.

Solutions

Have a "put away the day" activity. Have a little ritual where thoughts and worries are put away for the day. When a question or idea pops up during the routine, the parent can write it down on a little slip of paper and put it in a specially decorated box. You can tell your livewire that you'll answer or discuss these things tomorrow (and then make sure you do). This activity shows them that all the thinking and imagining and wondering for today is done. Nighttime is for resting the brain.

If you feel that your livewire needs a little more processing time, you could choose a moment way before bedtime when you recap the day. You could have set questions: What were the hard things that happened today? What awesome things happened today? What did you learn today that you didn't know before? (Make sure to end on the good things.) Write the answers down in a journal, then close it and put it away as a sign that it's time for the day's thinking to be done. If they bring any new thoughts up again during the routine, remind them that that's a "tomorrow thought" and maybe have them do this next activity.

Visualize letting go of thoughts until tomorrow. Once your talkative livewire is relaxed in bed, have them "see" their thoughts as balloons or bubbles. Give each thought a label like "recess" or "my new story idea" and then have them release them into tomorrow and watch them float away.

Don't feed the monkeys. Doing a lot of explaining or talking rarely, if ever, helps a talker stop talking. It just throws more fuel on the fire. If you know that responding with words—*"Okay, honey, it's time to go to sleep now because you are tired"*—just engages them more, start reducing the number of words you use. A simple "night-night" or "sleepy time" (or similar) as a response to everything they say will show your chatty livewire that the time for conversation is done and you are not going to be throwing the ball back. Once the light goes out, conversation should really stop.

The Mind Racer

Livewires are big and active thinkers. They pick up on everything, and as a result, their uber active, aware mind can run away with them, whether for good or ill. Smarts, sensitivity, and perceptiveness make livewires more vulnerable to a burst of creativity or worrying / overthinking just as the lights go out. Their thoughts start to ramp up, and because their level of awareness isn't tempered by experience, even small events can trip them up. They may not know that the tornado they saw on TV can't happen where they live. In their mind, if it happened *somewhere*, it could happen *anywhere*, and now they're worried about tornadoes. They may have new ideas for the story they're writing, or they're still wondering why that classmate abandoned them at recess.

I used to tell my daughter that her brain was like a powerful team of runaway horses, and she was holding the reins. She had to learn how to drive those powerful thought horses, so they didn't run away with her. Working on teaching your child how to calm their brain down when it starts running away can help bedtime, as well as give them skills for the long-term.

Solutions

Watch what they're exposed to. I don't need to tell you that livewires' mental antennae are always scanning for information. You have to be extra careful with these input sponges and what they might see on television or other sources of media. Livewires who are sensitive and perceptive are, by their nature, worriers and can be very, *very* easily thrown by things you might not think they would even notice . . . but they *do*. Sad, frightening, or just intense images or events impact sensitive livewires more profoundly—even at very young ages—and it can be difficult for them to easily bounce back. It's such a challenge, and it's so hard to prevent, I know. Where you can, monitor what they are watching (or what you are watching that they may see, even if it's just a commercial or an image that appeared before you were able to change the channel). Once they see something they shouldn't and begin to think about it, it's going to be harder to deal with than preventing it in the first place.

Your livewire may react even to images that are totally benign. Some of the totally normal, typical fears that young children have can be more subtle than monsters under the bed. The following fears are known to occur as a normal part of development at certain ages, as new understandings and cognitive abilities come online.[50]

Additionally, for young children, images in movies or television can trigger new fears. Joanne Cantor, author and researcher on the

AGE-APPROPRIATE FEARS

2 to 3 years	Animals The dark Thunder / lightning / loud noises People in costume Sounds outside their control (toilet flushing, barking dogs) Separation from parent
4 to 5 years	Bugs Getting lost Monsters Shadows Death
5 to 7 years	Germs / illness Natural disasters "Bad" people School

effects of media on young children's fears, lists some common media images that can also trigger fear in small children:

- Something that looks scary, even if it's benign (kind alien, silly monster)
- Supernatural events / people or magic (witches / wizards, spells / curses)
- Transformations (when one thing turns into another, like the Incredible Hulk)
- Real-life footage of tornadoes, hurricanes, floods, fires, etc.
- Sad images or stories (how many of us were scarred by *Bambi* or *Dumbo* back in the day?)[51]

It's important to remember that livewires can be ahead of the developmental game where fears are concerned, too. The downside of being a perceptive smarty-pants is that a young livewire can end up worried or frightened by snippets of events or bits of information that others don't even notice because, while livewires have the brainpower to pick up the information, they don't have the context to put it in perspective. They also can't let it go as easily as other children. They hear that a tornado happened *somewhere*, and think, *Wait, doesn't that mean it can happen <u>here</u>?* And now they're worried about tornadoes even though they don't happen where you live.

It may be impossible to fully insulate them from exposure to images that affect them. It's going to be important to have some strategies for addressing those fears.

Validate and refocus. Even if your fretful livewire is worried about something improbable or even impossible, validate that feeling worried is okay. Don't try to talk them out of it . . . especially *now*, at bedtime. Sometimes talking more about the worry (or why they shouldn't be worried) further inflates it. Acknowledge that they feel worried, then suggest that you talk more about it tomorrow. Move right away to helping them refocus on their just-as-real feelings of safety in their house and in their bed. Help them feel grounded in the present place and moment by feeling their body on the bed and the blankets on top of them. Try to focus on concrete input from their senses: What do they see? What do they hear? What do they feel? Validate, refocus, and ground—these techniques will come in handy anytime your livewire's brain starts spinning. Practice now while they're young.

Body-oriented calming. Sometimes the best way to calm the brain is to begin with the body. Bedtime yoga or other stretching and progressive relaxation strategies are great for overthinkers. Getting them in their bodies helps take focus away from their brain. If they are in bed with a runaway brain, ask them where they're feeling the overflow of thoughts or worries in their bodies. Then, have them mentally scan their body for places that need to be looser or calmer and have them breathe deeply into those places. You can help them use their imagination to send "love energy" or "calm energy" or even just a color to those places. Have them breathe deeply to change the color to something brighter or lighter. Tuning in to physical relaxation can really help that busy brain settle down.

The Mind Racer—Fear of the Dark Edition

Fear of the dark (or the monsters that might lurk within it) is a common issue for busy-brain livewires and one that can keep parents heavily involved in the go-to-sleep process. When children are afraid, our first impulse is to comfort them, and then try to tell them why they don't need to be afraid. All good . . . but it doesn't always work.

The latest thinking about anxieties and fears is that rather than accommodating them (turning on a light, staying until they're asleep), we need to help children gradually practice confronting small amounts of precisely what they're afraid of in a safe context. For example, if they're freaking out about being alone in their room at night (or ever), start with helping them practice being alone for tiny bits of time (count to ten?) during the day. Make it a game and give lots of positive reinforcement for any achievement.

Accommodating your child's fears by turning on a light or sleeping in the room with them can feel like a perfectly reasonable response (and it technically is). But it ultimately prevents the child from getting better at handling those fears.

Solutions for fear of monsters

Fear of monsters is a double-whammy of scary imaginative images and being alone in their room, and the age of the child will dictate how you approach these fears. Younger children (definitely under four, but really under seven) have not yet developed the ability to differentiate between real and imagined.[52] They may *know* that monsters are imaginary, but they also believe that what they imagine could become real.[53] This is why it doesn't help to say "monsters aren't real." So, at these early ages, "magical" strategies—monster repellant sprays, "Monsters Keep Out" signs, etc.— can help. These strategies give your livewire the power to keep the scary thing away.

You can also do a little fun reframing of what they're scared of.[54] Not all monsters are bad. Elmo and Grover are monsters, for example. Have them give their monster a funny or cute name like Daisy, Fred, or Gladys (full disclosure, I do this for spiders). Have them draw a picture of the monster with a silly expression or a funny hat.

Older children become increasingly capable of understanding that the scary shadow in their room is not a monster, it's just a shadow. This understanding is dependent on cognitive development. While some children will respond to reality checking ("monsters aren't real" or "that shadow isn't an alligator") starting at four, this skill isn't fully online until closer to seven.[55]

Solutions for fear of the dark

Fear of the dark is really fear of the unknown. So, if we can get the dark to be less unknown, it can potentially help reduce the fear.[56] If you stay with them every night or do things to prevent them from feeling fearful, they have no opportunity to get better at conquering this feeling. Instead, do some darkness detective work, maybe during Special Time. Give them a flashlight and have them show you all the parts of their room that are scary. Investigate them together. Does an object cast a scary shadow? Move or hide it. Does the open closet door seem creepy? Close it. (Experts call this strategy *reality affirmation*.)[57] Investigating the source of their dark-based fear helps mind racers develop the courage to challenge what they're afraid of and gain a little mastery over it.

I frequently recommend the following research-based games[58] that help children progressively get more comfortable with being in the dark. These are listed in order of how challenging they are. Once your livewire seems to be comfortable doing one game, you can move to the next one to up the stakes a little.

Blindfold game. Put a blindfold on your child and have them try to find large pieces of furniture or a toy in their room (make sure it's easily located). You can gradually make the toy harder to find. Make a big deal about it when they find it.

Toy-in-the-room game. Get your child to go into a dark room to get a toy from a specific place (for example, "Go get the pink teddy bear that's on your bed."). Again, give lots of praise when they do it.

Animal sounds game. Have the child lie on their bed in as much darkness as you think they can handle. You go sit in the hall or somewhere nearby and make an animal sound that they have to identify. Begin with easy sounds (no scary ones, of course) and gradually increase the time they have to wait for the next sound and/or how dark the room is.

Animals-on-the-wall game. Make animal hand shadows on the wall in their darkened bedroom.

Flip-the-switch game. When a parent yells "Go!" from the other room, the child in the bedroom gets up from the floor, turns off the light, and goes to lie in bed before the parent arrives to turn the light back on. Gradually lengthen how long they wait before the light is turned on.

Toy-in-the-dark game. This is similar to the toy-in-the-room game, except you place the toy somewhere and they have to look for it. (You don't have to make the toy challenging to find. Them just being in the dark is the point.)

Find-the-noisy-box game. The game begins in a totally dark house. Your child lies in their bed, and you shake a cereal box (or something else that makes a sound) from somewhere in the house. Your child has to go through the dark house, turning on lights to find you. You can gradually increase the difficulty of finding you or the time it takes between making the sound. Go as slowly as your child needs you to.

The key to working with nighttime fears is to tread the line between validating the feelings and challenging them to get better at confronting them. We're not serving our children by preventing or rescuing them from their worried or scared feelings (that's impossible, anyway). We have to help them practice getting better at coping with them.

The Holder-Toucher-Stroker-Cuddler

Some livewires seem to need a ton of sensory input at bedtime and once the lights are out: full body contact, holding hands, holding hair, patting eyelashes, putting their finger in your mouth (yup, we've both heard this one), stroking the parent's eyebrow (heard this one, too), etc. Not only can this be exhausting (and triggering) for a parent, but these behaviors do not usually shift on their own.

The most effective solution here is often substitution—swapping in something else for whatever *you*-centered tactile strategy your livewire currently has. To do this, you may need to get creative. The trick here is to look at what type of input your livewire seems to be needing as they're falling asleep and come up with a reasonable substitute. Can the fringe on a pillow (or the mane on a stuffed horse) substitute for hair? Can a body pillow substitute for your body next to them? I've had parents whose child held their hand to sleep put the hand in a glove and gradually, over a couple of days, slide their hand out so that the child was just holding the glove. I've also had parents stuff the glove, so it's more like a hand. I had one mom whose child had to stroke her eyebrow to fall asleep. We ended up finding her a little stuffed caterpillar that had bristles on it.

Think about whether there's something you can offer your child that could be a stand-in for whatever it is that they're currently depending on. An even better idea is to have your older livewire brainstorm with you. Kim worked with a mom whose daughter twirled mom's hair to sleep. She brought her daughter to a store and together they picked out a tassel for her to twirl at bedtime instead. You can also talk to your child about it. Ask *why* they like doing what they're currently doing and then talk to them about why it's not working for you. Then you can figure out a substitute together that works for everyone.

The magic of the Bedtime Chart

With livewires, you have to stay three steps ahead of them at all times . . . and *especially* at bedtime.

LIVEWIRE: I want to listen to an audio story.

TIRED PARENT: We said only two stories, and I've already read two.

LIVEWIRE: But I want to listen to the audio one. You didn't say anything about those.

You didn't see that one coming, did you? Livewires are *so smart*, and the number of curveballs they can throw at us at bedtime means that we constantly are making split-second, spur-of-the-moment, I'm-too-tired-to-fight-it decisions. You know that if you say yes, it's going to become something that has to happen every night. And if you say no, there will be a frustration meltdown fueled by bedtime fatigue. So fun.

The solution to this is a planned, set-in-stone Bedtime Chart. This is not a sticker chart. We are not going to have them work to earn some kind of future reward. Future rewards (*"If you earn seven stickers you will get a . . ."*) seldom work for livewires because you're asking them to give up something *now* for some theoretical future reward. Also, stickers just aren't always that motivating.

The Bedtime Chart is more like a contract for what will and won't happen. It's a premade, well-thought-out sequence of steps that you create and frequently review *with your livewire* that helps everyone understand what will and will not happen at night. This way, if a spur-of-the-moment curveball does get thrown (*"I'm hungry. I want a banana"*), you are prepared. You can carefully check the chart. (*"Hmm, let me see. Banana, banana . . . nope, I don't see anything here about a banana. Shoot. We'll talk about whether we should add having a snack to the chart tomorrow, but for tonight, no banana."*) Blame the chart if you have to.

Important rule: If it's not on the chart, it doesn't happen.

The key is to lock down openings for negotiation. You might be able to be a little more flexible in the future, but for right now while you're trying to establish some new patterns, the ground rules need to be pretty set in stone.

In Kim's first book, *The Sleep Lady's Good Night, Sleep Tight*, she calls this chart a Sleep Manners Chart. *Manners* refers to behaviors we expect to see or are working toward. The chart is not for earning stickers or having consequences. It's about helping everyone know what's expected at bedtime and during the night.

The chart doesn't have to be a major craft project. If you like crafts, go crazy, but it can also just be a document that you create with clip art and then print out as you need it (daily, weekly). You could even put the chart on a clipboard and make your livewire the "boss of the routine." I've heard of parents who act like they don't know what comes next and let their livewire tell them. This is another tool to give your livewire a teeny bit more of the control they're usually trying to get through stalling or cranking out a million requests.

WORKBOOK TO DO

Turn to the Bedtime Routine Worksheet in your Workbook and start thinking about what will be in your routine as you read the following sections. There are also Bedtime Chart examples.

Making the chart

Have a family meeting with your child *during the day* to craft the Bedtime Chart. What comes first? What do they *absolutely* need to go to sleep? How many books will be read? (You might need to set a maximum amount of reading time if they decide to poke the limit by picking two giant books.) Include line items for last snack, last drink of water, last trip to the bathroom, last moment to pick your stuffed animal, etc. Make sure to indicate which parent is doing Special Time and which parent is doing bedtime. (You could have pictures for both parents each night and just circle who is doing what.)

Also, if you are creating a weekly chart, remember to include space for any changes that may happen day-to-day or during a particular week. If there's an event coming up and a babysitter or grandparent will be there for bedtime instead, *put it in the chart.* You really don't want any surprises. If something can be anticipated and plugged into the chart, it should be. Try to be as detailed as you can in anticipating all the twists and turns your child may throw at you at bedtime.

Be sure to include post-lights-out shenanigan prevention. Even though we're talking about getting ready for saying good night and turning off the light, a preset plan also needs to include what you expect them to do *after* the lights are out. What's going to happen if they get out of bed after bedtime? What happens if they start goofing around or yelling? Decide ahead of time and stick to it.

- Do you want them in their bed all night?
- Is it okay if they co-sleep after a certain hour?
- Is it okay if they come into your room but sleep on a mattress on the floor (as long as they don't wake you up)?

Make sure to put your expectations on the chart and phrase them in terms of what you want them to do (as opposed to what you don't want them to do). Instead of writing "I don't get out of bed" (because a child only hears "get out of bed"), phrase it as "I stay in my bed once the lights are out."

You can also include a few line items describing *your* post-lights-out actions (we'll focus on this more in the next chapters). This can communicate that the chart is for everyone, not just your child. It also gives them some warning about what you will be doing (staying until they're asleep) and what you won't (having any more conversations). A few examples:

"I will sit in the chair until you are fully asleep."
"I will only use the word 'night-night' once the lights are out."
"I will check on you right before I go to bed."
"If you wake up, I will walk with you back to bed and then sit in the chair until you're back asleep."

Using the Bedtime Chart

Once you have crafted the chart and everyone knows what's on it, there are still a couple of preliminary steps to take before using it at bedtime.

Give them a heads-up. Go over the chart *during the day* and then again *before bedtime begins* to remind them about the sequence of steps and what you expect them to do. (Once they have really gotten the hang of the routine, you don't have to warn them anymore—but you can, if you think it helps.)

Rehearse bedtime changes during the day. If there are any new steps or adjustments to what you are doing at bedtime, try a rehearsal of it at some point during the day. For example, if you are not going to be lying down with them for the first time that night, have them get in bed and you sit next to their bed. Have them test drive this new setup. *"Okay, you get in bed and pretend like you're going to sleep. I'm going to sit here in the chair so you can see how that will be."* Or if you're okay with them coming into your room in the middle of the night, have them practice doing that quietly: *"Okay, you get in your bed and pretend to be asleep. I'll go in my room and pretend to be asleep. When I say 'Go,' see how quietly you can come into our room and get on your floor bed."* If you're using a wake-up clock for the first time, rehearse having it turn on or change color first before they come to your room. That way, you're practicing both skills—using the wake-up clock and coming into your room like a ninja.

Have your child experience what it's like so they can work out their resistance or worries while you're both still alert and awake. Invite them to ask questions or even (eek) suggest modifications. You can also prep them in other ways. I heard of a mom who made a picture book to show how everything at bedtime would go. You could do a run-through with little people or stuffed animals. Any method that gives them hands-on preparation for whatever will happen will prevent them from feeling blindsided or surprised at bedtime.

Check off steps as you go. This is an important step because you want to establish that the chart is the contract. Once something is checked off, it's done.

Review and assess the next day. The next morning, review the previous night. Make a big deal about any steps or behaviors the child did well. Really recognize *any* improvement and make the recognition focused on the behavior (*"Wow! You know what? You stayed in your bed for thirty minutes last night! That's ten minutes longer than the night before!"*). Play down (or maybe don't even mention) what didn't go so well. Parenting expert John Sommers-Flanagan calls this *reverse behavior modification.*[59] By focusing attention on what your child did *well*, you are encouraging them to do more of that. Young ones who may be on the receiving end of a lot of "don'ts" and "nos" during the day especially respond to this tactic. (A focus on what's working may also help *you* feel a little more positive. Bonus!)

If you feel like you need to comment on elements that are still works in progress, go lightly. Livewires can really take things in deeply (especially the perfectionistic ones). Maybe just briefly say, "Staying in bed was hard for you last night. Sometimes it just takes practice." And then leave it alone.

If you're going to use any rewards, base them on what your child has *already* done, rather than what they might do in the future. Rather than having a future-based incentive (*"If you get five stickers, you can have ice cream"*), do something to acknowledge what they've already achieved. Surprise them with a family ice cream outing, for example, because they improved three nights in a row. For daily improvements, you could offer a small treat or reward right away the next day. I worked with parents who would give one chocolate chip in the morning for a good night. It was a tiny thing and happened close in time to the child's efforts overnight. Use what you think will best help acknowledge their progress.

PUTTING IT ALL TOGETHER: WHAT'S IN YOUR ROUTINE?

Now that you have a variety of options that might work for your unique livewire at bedtime, start crafting your new routine. Let's summarize the elements we covered for a solid lead-up to lights out, by age.

Six Months to Almost Two Years
- If transitioning to a crib and/or a separate room, give your child time during the day to get acquainted with it.
- Check the sleep environment for distractions. Use blackout shades and white noise, and reduce visual clutter.
- Have a pre-routine routine. Lower the lights and turn off media before you even start the bedtime routine.
- Have a manageable, consistent routine that has at least one step after the final feed and before going into the crib. (For children older than a year, milk can be offered before the routine starts.)

Two Years
- Have a pre-routine routine. Schedule wind-down time before the routine begins (lower lights, turn on music, turn off screens). Decide if they need some physical wind down (stretching, etc.).
- Check the sleep environment for distractions. Use blackout shades and white noise.
- Have a manageable, very consistent routine with limits on how many options they have (books, drink of water, stuffed animals, etc.).
- Consider crafting a basic Bedtime Chart.

Three Years and Up
- Have a family meeting to craft a plan with your child and create a Bedtime Chart with the specific tasks and goals for bedtime.
- Rehearse any changes to their familiar routine ahead of bedtime.
- Have a pre-routine routine. Include steps for winding down ahead of starting the bedtime routine (Special Time, heavy work, yoga / stretching, mindfulness breathing, etc.).

- Check the sleep environment for distractions. Use blackout shades and white noise. Remove distracting toys or books.
- Have a consistent, manageable routine (that includes steps for calming mind and body) with no room for negotiation.
- Review the Bedtime Chart before bedtime. Check off steps as you go.
- Review the chart the next morning. Make a big deal over what went well and encourage practice for what is still a work in progress.

Once you are fully prepped with a solid pre-lights-out foundation, we are going to start on the work of shifting your child's sleep patterns so they have a clear road map for how to go *to* sleep and *back to* sleep with less and less help from you. But you don't have to jump into working on sleep right this minute. You may have found some changes in this chapter that you want to make *before* you dive into the big stuff. Is there anything (like making and using the Bedtime Chart, starting Special Time, etc.) that you want to start implementing *before* working on sleep skills? That's awesome. Just be sure to adjust your chart when you add those other pieces (where you'll be sitting, what you'll do once the lights go out, etc.).

Ready to move on to Big Strategy #3: Changing your child's go-to-sleep pattern? Let's turn the page!

OUR TRIP CHECKLIST

- ☑ You know you are on a different path.
- ☑ You understand your livewire's temperament strengths and challenges.
- ☑ You understand the link between temperament and sleep issues.
- ☑ Your child is ready:
  - ☑ Over six months
  - ☑ No upcoming disruptions
  - ☑ No physiological issues that affect sleep
- ☑ You are ready (or as ready as you can be).
- ☑ You understand the Big Four sources of sleep issues.

- ☑ Big Strategy #1: You know how to avoid that second wind.
- ☑ Big Strategy #2: You have a solid, consistent bedtime routine.
- ☐ Big Strategy #3 and #4: You know how to change the go-to-sleep and back-to-sleep patterns and are prepared to be more consistent than you've ever been before.
- ☐ You know how to track progress.
- ☐ You know how to diagnose and fix any problems that arise.
- ☐ BETTER SLEEP!

Rubber, Meet Road

CHAPTER 9

Big Strategies #3 and #4: Change the Go-to-Sleep Pattern (and Don't Turn Back)

Crafting Your Sleep Plan and Hitting the Road

Now that you have laid a great foundation with a full (or nearly full) nap tank, a well-timed bedtime, an effective transition, and a solid, unwavering bedtime routine, you are ready to start thinking about and planning for what needs to change about how your child currently falls asleep. This is where the rubber really meets the road. In this chapter, we're going to walk you through a new way to think about sleep patterns and how to make a solid plan for what needs to change and how you want to tackle it.

A LESS SHAME-Y WAY TO THINK ABOUT SLEEP

Too much of the advice around sleep training talks about breaking bad habits—like you've intentionally or out of permissiveness created the problem you're trying to confront. How sleep happens right now is neither good nor bad. If it's working, there's no problem. And if it's not working or is not sustainable, you can change it. No one needs to feel bad or wrong for it. Let's just make some adjustments to how you're approaching sleep so that it works better for everyone.

We're going to look at the process of going to sleep as a pattern or a script. The way sleep happens now is how your baby thinks all humans fall asleep. Older kiddos develop familiar patterns that they prefer. I mean, why wouldn't they want a parent to lie down with them and rub their back? It's a lovely, easy way to fall asleep. Although it's tempting to think that these patterns will change by themselves, they really don't. A child is not, one day—out of the blue—going to think, *I don't need that feeding / rocking / back rub to sleep anymore. I'll just do it myself.* But let's not call it a bad habit or a negative sleep association. It's just a pattern. Patterns can be changed anytime they stop working. No need to "break" anything.

HERE WE GO: THE BIG SLEEP TRAINING SECRET NO ONE WANTS YOU TO KNOW

It may seem like there are dozens of completely unique sleep training methods out there, and you just have to find the right one to have success. But here's the *big sleep training secret* that no one says out loud. They all boil down to *one* simple action:

Change the pattern.

That's it. That's the whole deal. The goal of *any* method for working on sleep is to shift the go-to-sleep pattern from *you* doing the work of getting your child sleep to *your child* doing almost all of it. The only real difference between methods has to do with how much support or soothing you're allowed to give your child—no support (cold turkey, pure extinction), minimal support (Ferber, graduated extinction), or tons of support (the Sleep Lady Shuffle / chair method, no-cry strategies)—and how present you are—leave the room (Ferber, cold turkey, pop-ins, etc.) or stay in the room

(Sleep Lady Shuffle, "pick up, put down," etc.). They *all* are variations on the same core task: changing the go-to-sleep pattern.

It would be great if, instead of having to sleep coach, we could just have a conversation with our livewire and tell them how to go to sleep: *"Okay, child. To go to sleep, you lie down, close your eyes, and just relax. Then you fall asleep!"* Instead, all we can do is *show* them by altering what we do (*all* the work) to something new (*less* of the work) in a methodical and consistent way.

Here's an overview of how we're going to do that:

1. **Give them a new go-to-sleep pattern at bedtime that doesn't rely on feeding / bouncing / lying down with them.** We want them doing most of the go-to-sleep work.

2. **Provide lots of presence and support at first** while they are wrestling with and adjusting to the new pattern and then back that support off gradually over time.

3. **Be as consistent as humanly possible** so that the new pattern is clear enough for them to detect and practice it.

4. **Push all the way through on those bumpy first couple of days.** You will need to muscle through at least a few days of pushback to get those patterns to budge.

5. **Be super kind to yourself and patient with the process.**

THE CRITICAL IMPORTANCE OF BEDTIME FOR CHANGING PATTERNS

Bedtime is the most important moment for working on sleep because it's the best time for helping your child shift familiar go-to-sleep patterns. You are awake and alert (mostly), and your child has that evening release of melatonin and a push of sleep pressure.

Bedtime also establishes *the template* for how your child thinks that sleep happens. *"I'm fed, I'm held (or Mom / Dad is rubbing my back) . . . aaaand I'm asleep."* So, when they wake up at night and they're suddenly in the crib / bed alone, they're going to wonder how the heck they got there.

They're also not going to know how to get *back* to sleep without a repeat of their bedtime go-to-sleep pattern.

I've had lots of parents who are doing whatever is necessary to get their child all the way to sleep at bedtime but expect them to be able to go back to sleep in the middle of the night on their own. Their child has no idea what to do because the bedtime template looks different. For them, sleep happens because of feeding / holding / back rubbing. They don't know that there's another way.

So, we start with bedtime, and introduce a new way.

Once a child is aware of where they are as their eyes close and they've done most if not all the work to get there, then they have a road map for what to do when they wake at night. You will no longer be a necessary part of their go-to-sleep template, so you will not be a necessary part of their back-to-sleep template, either.

> **The go-to-sleep pattern *creates a little breadcrumb trail that a child can use to get back to sleep when they wake at night.***

Shifting this pattern to one that is more independent is really the only way to facilitate better, longer sleep. There's honestly no way around that. But don't worry. We've already done a lot that will set you up for success, and we're going to make sure that you feel as clear and confident as possible so you can feel good about the road ahead.

DECISIONS TO MAKE BEFORE WE CREATE YOUR PLAN

Before we begin, there are a few more decisions you will need to make before getting started.

WORKBOOK TO DO

Go to the Change the Pattern Worksheet in the Workbook. As you read the following sections, make notes about what you plan to do.

How much of the night do you think you can take on?

Consistency is going to be one of the most important ingredients of success in this journey. So, it's important to really know your limits. You don't have to tackle bedtime *and* the whole night if you just don't have enough gas in your tank. Figure out how much of the work you *know* you can take on. Can you *only* manage working on bedtime? Bedtime and any wake-ups until you go to bed? Wake-ups until midnight? Bedtime and all night until 5 AM?

Working on part of the night means that you will be doing what you usually do for the rest of the night. The whole process may take longer, but this is a fine choice if you are really exhausted.

> *It's okay to pick your battles—but*
> *fight the ones you pick.*

Remember, consistency is critical. If you take on more than you have the emotional or physical reserves for, you won't have enough stamina to withstand your livewire's unavoidable pushback. The result will be inconsistency or just throwing in the towel. We don't want that. Take on only as much as you can really, really commit to. If you can only do bedtime, just do *that*. Then, once you see a little success at bedtime, you'll feel more motivated to tackle wake-ups.

Who will do what?

We don't recommend that one parent take on the whole night, if two parents (or a parent and another caregiver) are available. If at all possible, this is a two-person job. Even if one partner has a more intense job, it's reasonable to share this load and the temporarily broken sleep it comes with for a few weeks. An adult can function adequately on a five-hour block of sleep, at least long enough to sleep coach. This is all-hands-on-deck time.

There are a variety of ways to divide the work of bedtime and night-time. You could split up the night with one parent doing bedtime and all wake-ups until midnight or so, and the other parent taking the rest of the night. You could have one parent do everything for a while and then introduce the other partner in a few days. You could even switch off days. There's no right or wrong. Just make sure that whoever is doing most of the coaching on one night can get a little rest the next day.

If one parent has been mostly in charge of bedtime and nighttime until now, starting to sleep coach can be a moment for the other parent to really shine (especially if the current sleep routine is centered around nursing). A new person doing bedtime signals a brand-new routine or approach to sleep: new person, new pattern. We suggest having this parent do bedtime and as many wake-ups as possible for the first couple of days. You might also decide to do the current routine together for a few days leading up to the start of sleep coaching. This gives your livewire some time to wrap their head around the possibility of another person participating in bedtime.

When you do decide to fold the original parent back in, there can be a bump *up* in protest or wakefulness (especially if that partner was nursing or rocking your child to sleep). Your livewire may think, *Finally! Whew! We're going back to the way it used to be!* and then be a teeeeny bit irked that it's not. That's okay. It takes time to acclimate to new patterns. We should expect them to be a little thrown.

The key to having two parents doing this successfully is coordination and consistency. Try to make absolutely sure that, no matter who's doing the work, the *same thing* happens so that the pattern stays uber consistent. Too much discrepancy can throw off progress because your sharp little livewire will see that there's wiggle room between the two of you and jump on it hard. Once they understand that nothing changes based on who's in the room, they will—eventually—settle into the new way of getting to sleep.

Where is square one?

Because you have a livewire, we're not going to assume that your starting line is the same as ours. Generally, the first step of sleep coaching starts with you putting your livewire into the crib or bed *awake*. If you have been co-sleeping full-time or doing *a lot* of rocking, bouncing, or lying with your child, putting them right into bed awake might be too massive a change. You will need to figure out what *your* square one is going to be. You may need to spend some time with training wheels on before you have them hop onto the two-wheeler.

If you have been bouncing your livewire *all the way* to sleep, for example, you may need to take a few days to first work on bouncing slower and slower until you can successfully stop bouncing. Or, if you have been lying with your livewire, letting them use you as their body pillow, you may want to spend a few nights introducing an actual body pillow or new stuffed animal for them to cuddle. Taking just a couple of extra days to ease into the new pattern can help unadaptable, intense livewires get ready for the changes that are coming. However, for some livewires, *any* change is a big deal and baby steps are just as hard as big ones. If this is true for your child, you may want to skip the training wheels and make changes all at once on Day One.

Forging New Go-to-Sleep /
Back-to-Sleep Patterns

Okay, friends, deep breath, here we go.

The approach we're going to use to change your livewire's sleep patterns was created and pioneered over twenty years ago by Kim, who calls it the Sleep Lady Shuffle (aka the Shuffle or SLS). In research circles, it's called *parental fading* or a *responsive approach*. I've heard parents also refer to it as the *chair method* (though in some places, it's described inaccurately). This approach has been shown to be as effective as cry it out, less physiologically stressful,[60] and much more tolerable for both parents and children (even the intense ones).

This approach works so well because it's consistent with how we teach children nearly every other new skill: We help them a lot at first. Then, we let them practice doing more and more on their own. You don't show a child a two-wheeler and say, "Good luck with this, kiddo. I'll be inside. If I help you, you won't learn to do it yourself." No. You hold tightly on to the back of the seat until the child starts getting a feel for it. Then, you start *gradually* letting go—with a hand hovering right behind to catch the bike if it starts tipping over. The better the child gets at balancing, the more you let go. We're going to do the same thing for sleep. You get to start out right there with them, and then, as they get the hang of things, we are going to start gradually reducing how much you are doing and how close you are to them as they are falling asleep. Makes sense, doesn't it?

In this chapter, we're going to break down this approach into very straightforward pieces that apply to all kiddos regardless of their age or where they're sleeping. Then, in the following two chapters, we'll give specific details for two age subgroups. Chapter ten will address infants / toddlers under three (mostly in cribs) and chapter eleven will cover livewires three and up (mostly in beds).

Feel free to use your best judgment about which chapter applies best to your livewire. There are some two-and-a-half-year-olds in a bed who can handle the strategies suggested for three-year-olds. Pick whatever's going to work best for your livewire, the layout of your house, the needs of your family, etc. For families who are co-sleeping or using a floor bed, or who have a little crib escape artist who needs to be in a bed, we'll cover adjustments that you can make to accommodate those realities. The process is modifiable for different families in different contexts. Remember, there are many right ways for sleep to happen. Isn't that good news?

THE NUTS AND BOLTS OF THE SHUFFLE

The Shuffle is really simple . . . at least to explain. The basic premise is that, while your child learns how to fall asleep in the crib or bed on their own, you're going to offer a lot of support and help. Then you're going to gradually reduce that help over time. Remember the ultimate goal: **to transfer the work of going to sleep from mostly *you* to mostly *them***.

AN OVERVIEW OF THE SHUFFLE

- Get your livewire in the crib / bed ready for sleep but *awake*.
- Sit in a chair right beside the crib / bed.
- Give intermittent help / support / encouragement at first while they learn a new go-to-sleep pattern, calming them down when they need it.
- Do this until they're completely asleep.
- Every time they wake up (if it's not a feed time), do the same thing until they're back asleep.
- Over the course of two(ish) weeks, move farther away from their cribside / bedside every few days.

The first step of the Shuffle as written starts out with you sitting in a chair beside your livewire's crib or bed. Remember, you can start from wherever your square one is. Maybe your Day One will be rocking them to sleep instead of nursing. Or maybe it's lying with your toddler as they get used to falling asleep without the pacifier. Or maybe it's bouncing slower on the yoga ball for a few days, then sitting on the ball without bouncing, *then* moving to the crib.

No matter where you need to start or how small the changes need to be, just make sure you remember the driving idea of the Shuffle:

**Whatever you choose to do, always
be moving toward doing less.**

Let's start by going through the basic elements of the Shuffle, which apply to all ages and sleep situations. It's important to understand the basic structure because, first, it's surprisingly simple, and second, once you understand it, you will be able to modify it and use it in a way that fits you and your livewire. Ready? Here we go!

Days One to Three: Position One

BEDTIME: SIT IN A CHAIR (OR ON THE FLOOR) RIGHT BESIDE THE CRIB / BED

After you have done all your pre-bedtime prep (pre-routine, routine, etc.), you are going to get your livewire into bed, ready for sleep but awake. (Not "drowsy but awake." *Awake.*) We want them learning to go the whole way to sleep at bedtime so they understand how to get back to sleep under their own steam when they wake at night. You are going to sit in a chair (or on the floor) *right next to the crib or bed*. While they grapple with what in the world you are asking them to do (spoiler alert: they're going to cry), you can *intermittently* pat them, shush them, hum, rub their back / tummy, etc., until they're totally asleep. (I feel your skepticism. Hang on.)

The intermittent part is important. Anything you are doing the *whole* time can get unintentionally knitted into the new pattern. You don't want that. You want to do enough to let them know that you're there and helping but not so much that you accidentally become a part of their new template for sleep. It's like we're saying, "Here's a compromise: I'll be right here to support you and encourage you and help you, but I'm not going to do the work for you."

The fine line between "helping" and "doing too much" is not always clear, and you may have to do some careful testing: Are you responding too much? Or is it keeping them out of full-on freak-out? You may need to experiment to find out what that line is. You will not derail the process by missing the mark once or twice. (We're going to talk later about how to know if you've actually gone off the rails, I promise.)

We also want you to, as Kim says, "control the touch"—meaning, don't let them grab your hand (or hair or shirt). Instead, put your hand on top of or around theirs and make sure that you are in control, so you can make sure the touch really is off and on. Be careful not to let them fall asleep while holding your hand or finger. Remember, whatever they're doing as they're falling asleep is what they're going to try to re-create in the middle of the night. You don't want your hand (finger / ear / eyelashes / eyebrow) to accidentally get knitted into their go-to-sleep pattern.

It's also important to reduce how much touching / patting / stroking you are doing each day, *if you can*, because on Day Four, you're going to be moving out of touching distance. If your starting point requires a TON of touching (because just getting them in bed awake was a huge lift), you can add an extra day to this first position to taper down the patting / handhold-ing, etc., so that the jump to "no touching" is a little less stark.

It's important for us to say:

You cannot make a "deal-breaker" mistake here.
Try not to worry about getting it exactly right.

There's a learning curve, so cut yourself some slack. There are going to be curveballs. Just keep putting one foot in front of the other.

If they really lose it, you get to pick
them up to calm them down.

This is where the Shuffle is massively different from other methods. In most sleep training approaches, helping a child calm down is seen as a bad thing. If you've already tried those other methods, I'm pretty sure you found out quickly that once your livewire got going, there was not going to be any "self-soothing" going on. With the Shuffle, you can step in and help them calm down *at any point that you think your livewire is getting to their upper limit of okay.* For livewires in cribs, you get to pick them up to help calm them. For little ones in a bed, you can give them a hug or a drink of water. Here's the catch: Once they're calm, get back up on the horse and keep going . . . even if they start freaking out again. That's okay. We're going to keep helping them calm down and then continuing on.

NIGHTTIME WAKE-UPS: DO THE SAME THING YOU DID AT BEDTIME

If you have decided to also work on some or all wake-ups at night, you're going to go back to the spot you were in at bedtime and do *exactly the same thing* to get them back to sleep. (For those of you with babies still feeding at night, in the next chapter we're going to talk about how to handle planned night feeds versus other wake-ups.) You want your livewire to get the message that no matter when they wake up (and no matter who's attending to them), the *same thing* is going to happen. If we introduce unknowns (*"Will I get to co-sleep? Will I get rocked? Will they try for a while to get me back to sleep and then do what we used to do?"*), improvement can stall—or not happen at all. The key is *consistency, consistency, consistency* across all go-to-sleep and back-to-sleep moments.

If you've decided to work on bedtime only or bedtime and just a few of the wake-ups, that's okay. Even though your response won't be exactly the same across the whole night, you will be working on bedtime and giving a little practice during the wake-ups you've chosen to work on. In this scenario, you will be consistent within your planned timeframe (for example, bedtime and all wake-ups before 11 PM). We just want to avoid *unpredictable* inconsistency where, from the child's perspective, it's different every time they wake up.

A WORD ABOUT USING SCREENS WHILE YOU SIT WITH YOUR CHILD

While we know that sitting in the dark waiting for your nonsleepy livewire to fall asleep can be astonishingly boring, be judicious about getting too engrossed in your phone. The key to staying with your child is your presence but also your *emotional availability*. Research from the University of Pennsylvania found that parents' emotional availability at bedtime directly resulted in better sleep.[61] If you're *physically* present but mentally or emotionally not, your astute, perceptive child is going to notice (and maybe work harder to get your attention, which we do not want). Try listening to a podcast or book on tape instead of scrolling in the dark.

STAYING THE COURSE

Here's that game-changing information for livewires we promised you. If you've read any of the other books on sleep, you know their sleep advice essentially ends with "If you just do A, B, and C, in just a couple of nights—ta-da! Your child is sleeping through!" For livewires, there's way more to it.

The first few nights are where nearly all the hard work happens. In order to successfully navigate your way through, you're going to need some additional information and insight specific to livewires. There are some common road hazards in these first few nights that have likely derailed parents of persistent sleep fighters before. Let's make sure that doesn't happen to you.

First night real talk: It's going to be a rodeo.

Let's just agree that the first night is going to be a doozie. I'm not going to sugarcoat it. This first night, your child will be massively thrown. They have no idea what you are doing or why, and they do not like it one bit. They also don't know what you're expecting *them* to do.

"*Wait a gosh-darned minute! What's this nonsense? This isn't what we usually do! What are you expecting me to do here? I have no idea what I'm supposed to do! What the heck are you up to?*"

They *will* notice the discrepancy between this (which they don't like) and what you've been previously doing (which they do), and it's going to fry their circuits a little (or a lot). The first night's pushback can be big, and pushing through may take a while. There will likely be a moment where you *for sure* think that it's not working—but whatever you do, don't give up now. I call bedtime on Day One the first pancake. First pancakes are those little testers that always get tossed: too pale, too dark, shaped funny. The next ones are always better. So, set a low bar, expect it to look like it's not working, try to trust that it is, and move on to Day Two.

It's this first bit of freak-out that has caused many (most?) parents of livewires who have tried previous methods to stop after just *one* night of epic outrage. "*Well, we're not doing that again!*" Pushing through on this first night is absolutely key because we want and expect the second night to be better. (Livewire curveball caveat: If Day One was suspiciously easy, Day Two could be the rodeo. "*Wait, this nonsense is going on for more than one night? Um, no.*") Once you've made sure that there's nothing big standing in the way of sleep and you know that you have set your kiddo up for success, then you have to be ready for them to be confused and frustrated and maybe really hate the change. They're smart and vocal, and they're going to let us know about their displeasure with this new thing we're springing on them.

You have to push through the pushback.

This may sound daunting—and we get it. We *really, really* do. But you absolutely have to *push through* on these first few nights because, really, what's the alternative? If you have picked up this book, chances are that nothing is working right now—or it's kind of working but sucking the life out of you.

> **You can't sneak up on a livewire. There's nothing you can change that they won't notice.**

Anything you change is going to produce protest. They will clock even the tiniest alteration in your actions, and they will let you know that they do not like it one little bit. In other words, there will be drama, and that's okay.

Remember, while crying *will* happen, here's where the Shuffle differs from nearly all other sleep methods:

> **You are right there with them, and you can help them calm down whenever they need it.**

This is a whole different ball game from leaving them alone to figure it out. Research has found that parental presence during times of distress *reduces* children's physiological stress levels (and yours, too) even when they're crying.[62] We're going to make sure this period of freak-out doesn't go on very long. In chapter twelve, we will show you how to assess progress so that you don't have this much drama for too long. So, just hang in there for these first few days.

Don't turn back: Clarity, consistency, and commitment

Difficulty staying as consistent as you need to be with livewires is a huge reason why many parents' first attempts fail and why subsequent attempts may be even worse. Livewires put up an epic fight, and parents just don't have the stamina to battle as long as their livewire can (I mean, seriously). Parents of livewires are also in a near-constant state of self-doubt. Without a solid plan that you feel good about, it's common to have nagging doubts. *"What if I'm doing it wrong? Maybe this isn't the right thing to do. I wonder if I should have done that other thing first?"* You are now crafting a plan that feels tolerable for you and, while not fun, will also be tolerable for your livewire's temperament and level of development. Allow yourself to feel confident that this is a plan you can really commit to.

Consistency and commitment are the secret sauce of sleep coaching success. Babies learn through repetition, and smarty-pants toddlers learn through consistency that a new pattern is immune to their strategies.

This is especially true once you move to a new stage of the Shuffle. *You need to keep moving.* Don't do less, then go back to doing a little more, then less again. Once you stop a behavior (like patting) or you've moved away from lying down with them, *don't go back.* This is a common trap for parents. With livewires, we have to be crystal clear with our actions. Lack of clarity and consistency on your part means the new pattern is going to be harder for your livewire to pick up on. And if the pattern gets confusing, they are going to sit down in the middle of this new path we're on and refuse to budge. This needs to be a one-way road for a while: no U-turns, no detours.

The million-dollar question: How long do I try these first few nights?

Here's the hard answer: *as long as it takes.* Especially the first night (but, really, *all* nights).

I know, I *know.* It sounds terrifying. But during those first few nights, it's going to be critical that you push *all the way through.* Here's why (and this is a biggie): If you work and work and then say, "This is ridiculous. It's not happening. We'll just start again fresh tomorrow," you will not be starting "fresh." You won't be starting back at square one—you'll be starting from square negative ten.

Remember, there's very little you can sneak by your observant, mind-like-a-steel-trap child. Because you ended last night's coaching efforts with a "cookie" (what you used to do in the old pattern), you have inadvertently set the bar for how long they will fight you the next time you try. You have essentially said that nursing or rocking or lying down with you is *somewhere* on the table as an option, and they just have to find it. As persistent as these little ones are, we do *not* want to give them a reason to fight any harder than they're already going to.

Once you decide that you are going to start sleep coaching, you will need to really commit to pushing through for at least two or three days to see if sleep patterns will budge. I can't say this emphatically enough:

> **Pick what you know you can do and just . . .
> do . . . that . . . as consistently as humanly
> possible for at least two or three days.**

If you see any change at all, keep going. In chapter twelve, we will talk about what to do if you aren't getting *any* traction in these first few days. Do your very best to give it a solid push in Days 1 to 3. I promise we won't let you work for days and days with no improvement.

How long is "long" exactly?

It's hard to say, of course, but in our combined years of coaching, we would say that ninety minutes is on the upper end (could be a longer, could also be shorter). I've seen a few kids go two hours but not very many. I know this sounds difficult, but hopefully, these first couple of days are the biggest hills you'll have to climb.

What if it's longer than that? This is a fair question. It's also an area where it's difficult to give definitive advice. I certainly don't want any kiddo (or their parent) struggling and hysterical for hours and hours. I can't tell you to keep going if it's been three or four hours and your livewire isn't calming down or isn't going to sleep. That's a tall order for anyone. I would budget the two hours, and if you're going way past that with no signs of your child relenting, I'm going to give you permission to decide what to do next. In chapter twelve, we talk about what could be going on and how to make adjustments or pivot to see if that brings the freak-out level back down.

Here's a happy thought: Your livewire may completely surprise you and get on board much more quickly than you ever expected. This *does* sometimes happen because livewires are nothing if not unpredictable. Sometimes, when I work with parents, we're all prepared for the first-night rodeo—and then it ends up going *way* smoother than the parents expected. Sometimes, in less than a week, a sleep-allergic firecracker is sleeping through the night, and the parents wonder why they waited so long to work on sleep.

> *If you have noticed that all the usual go-to tricks*
> *have stopped working, that can be a sign that*
> *your livewire is ready to learn new sleep skills.*
> *It's possible this will go better than you think.*

Maybe expect it to be rough and then be grateful if it's not.

Isn't this just like cry it out?

While there *is* crying happening in this approach, there are a couple of important differences between this and cry it out. In those other methods, parents leave the room for set periods of time and only come in to *check* on their baby, not pick them up or fully soothe them. Parents are allowed to stay for only thirty seconds or so. Livewires can *really* lose it, and a parent only briefly popping in may not help much at all, which means, with cry it out, a child can end up staying in that hysterical state until they fall asleep (or don't). With the Shuffle, you are there with them the whole time, and you're allowed to bring them back to calm. We're never leaving them to cry intensely by themselves.

When we're right there, they're not crying because they're feeling scared or abandoned. They're just frustrated and confused. They don't know why we changed the routine or what we're expecting them to do. Crying *itself* isn't bad. It's the context, and how long a child is left in a highly distressed state without help or parents' presence.

They might also cry because this new approach is more work for them. Being fed and rocked to sleep is lovely and easy. Learning a new skill is work. Imagine for a minute that there was a pill that allowed you to eat whatever you wanted while remaining lean and strong. If I took that pill away and told you that you now had to go to the gym to achieve the same results, you wouldn't be happy. The gym is more work. The pill was so much easier. You'd probably cry, too, at the thought of having to go to the gym.

Of course, they're going to cry. We're changing their familiar patterns, and because they're babies, we can't warn them or explain the change to them. Your perceptive, change-averse livewire is going to hate this at first.

However, if you know that how things are *now* is not working or sustainable, you can't let the likelihood of big pushback stop you. There is no moment when their sleep challenges will just disappear. There will *never* be a time when they will gracefully (and silently) agree to fall asleep without help or without you in the room. They will not just "give up" a night feed. That's not how livewires roll. So, we will make sure to set them up for success, give them our presence and support, and then ask them to change their behavior a little so that they don't have zombies for parents.

ARE WE THERE YET? TRACKING PROGRESS

The first few days can be hard. There is no way around that. However, if you are 100 percent sure that your current situation needs to change, we encourage you to give it just three days or so to see if your new efforts result in any improvements in sleep. If they *do*, you should then see some really *big* changes (not resolution, but changes) in about a week (give or take).

Once you start coaching, make sure you're keeping track of your livewire's sleep with a sleep log. A sleep log doesn't have to be fancy. There's a blank Sleep Log template in your Workbook, but you can use an app or even just a blank piece of paper. Just make sure you keep track of the following:

- What time they were up for the day
- When naps were and how long they were
- What time bedtime was
- How long it took for your livewire to fall asleep
- How many wake-ups they had, at what time(s), how long they were, and what both you and your livewire did

This log is going to help you see progress when it may not be totally obvious. It'll also help you make connections between daytime sleep, bedtime strategies, and nighttime sleep patterns. If there's a night when sleep was unusually bad, for example, you can look at your log and see if nap timing or amount was off or if bedtime was too late. A log will also help you detect improvement, which is critical feedback for you.

It's important to keep in mind that *any improvement counts*. Let's say on Day One, your livewire screamed for ninety minutes and then woke every hour and a half all night (yikes, yes?). That's pretty awful. If on Day Two the freaking out was more off and on or less intense at bedtime and only lasted an hour, but they still woke up just as much, that's actually a shift. In this instance, I would say, "Let's keep going and see." We're looking to see if distress is less intense, less constant, or less long, and/or if there are fewer or shorter wake-ups and/or moments when you hear your child wake up and then go back to sleep. Those are all good signs that *something* is happening, and you should do a little happy dance.

I have had parents stop before Day Three, but only when (1) we already suspected something physical could be driving the sleep problems, and (2) Days One and Two were so bad that I couldn't make them go through one more night. These instances are really rare. If this is the case for you, reread chapter four to see if any of the physiological roadblocks are present. Otherwise, if you see any improvement, even if it's small, keep going.

Days Four to Six: Position Two

BEDTIME: MOVE YOUR CHAIR A FEW FEET AWAY FROM THE CRIB / BED AND USE ONLY YOUR VOICE TO SOOTHE

>> *For kids over three years old in beds, you can skip this position and move straight to Position Three, with the chair right to the door. Kim finds that this middle position can be too hard for kiddos in beds. However, if you feel like an interim step is going to work better for your livewire in a bed, keep reading.*

On Day Four, you are going to move your chair away from the crib / bedside. You can still always return to the crib or bed to pick up your child or hug them to calm them down if needed, but that will be it for physical contact: no more intermittent patting or touching.

It's common for there to be a bump up in protest on the fourth night of coaching. Why? This is your first move (another big change), and your livewire may make one last attempt to get things to go back to how they were. So, if the fourth night seems worse, don't worry. It's expected, and it's temporary. Don't let it throw you. Just . . . keep . . . going.

If you're having the impulse to go back to the crib or bed to pat or touch a lot even after moving away, you may need one more day at crib / bedside to really reduce your physical soothing before moving away again.

NIGHTTIME WAKE-UPS: DO THE SAME THING YOU DID AT BEDTIME

When your livewire wakes in the middle of the night, do a quick bedside / cribside check—make sure they don't have a fever, a diaper blowout, a foot stuck in their crib railing, etc. Once you're sure all is well and they're just frustrated, return to your chair. Stay until they're back asleep.

STAYING THE COURSE

Remember, these first few days are the hardest. Day Four is the first change you are making so it's important to really stick to the plan.

You have to make a move.

The three-day rule is important. I've had parents still sitting beside the crib or bed on Day Five or Six who wonder why things aren't improving. A really important part of this process is that you have to keep moving the goal line for your livewire. If you're in any one position for more than a few days, it becomes the new pattern, and suddenly you're starting from Day One all over again. Even if you've decided to use tiny little baby steps—keep moving!

Soothing should still be intermittent.

Even though you're just using your voice, you should still make sure you aren't singing (or whatever) the *whole* time. Anything you are consistently doing as they fall asleep becomes part of their new pattern. Even vocal soothing needs to be off and on, and you should be working to taper it down as the days go on.

Make sure "away" is away.

Be careful to avoid going back to the crib / bed for any reason other than picking your child up to calm them once you have moved away. That one extra hug, few more pats on the back, or brief head rub can seem so inconsequential, but it's a subtle, sneaky progress buster. It's not that touching is bad; it's just that in the first part of the sleep coaching process, it's super easy for tiny actions like these to become a new required component of the go-to-sleep pattern.

Both Kim and I have seen cases where progress has stalled, and when we ask what's happening at bedtime, a parent says, "I'm sitting in the chair away from the bed, and if I give them just one last head rub, they calm down and go right to sleep." If you are doing that "one little thing" consistently, it can get encoded in the pattern. Remember, livewires don't miss *a thing*, so the pattern *has* to be crystal clear. As much as humanly possible, once you move away from the crib / bed, try to keep pick-up-to-calm the only touching that happens.

A NOTE OF CAUTION

If you have picked your livewire up to calm them down and they promptly fall asleep on your shoulder, next time wait a moment or two longer before you pick them up.

Watch out for using too many words.

For verbal livewires, words will wake their brain right up. You don't need to do a lot of explaining (or even speak in full sentences) once the lights are out. Even for preverbal livewires, try to use just "night-night" or "time for sleep." If you must say anything, keep it brief.

COMMON WHAT IFS AT THIS POSITION

"What if we don't have a separate bedroom? How do we 'move away' when we're all in the same room?"

If your livewire needs to sleep in your room, progressively "moving away" at bedtime isn't an issue. You can follow the positions we'll outline here. The middle of the night is where you may need to get creative because you are right there in your bed. Consider using a room divider or privacy tent so that you and your livewire are at least visually separate. You may need to devise ways to keep doing less from where you're sleeping, such as spacing out how often you give verbal support from bed or reducing the volume of your vocalizing.

We also suggest potentially having one partner sleep in the living room during coaching, so both parents don't wake up every time your livewire does.

"What if their room is really small? If I move away, I'm already at the door."

Not every house or room allows for the chair locations that we outline in the Shuffle. If "away" is already "at the door" (Position Three) that's okay. You can just skip Position Two.

ARE WE THERE YET? TRACKING PROGRESS

I really wish I could tell you exactly how much improvement to expect at this stage. That would be *awesome*. Livewires, however, are difficult to predict.

In general, as long as you still see behaviors moving and changing (even if different things are changing each time), that's a good sign. Livewires don't improve in a straight line. I've seen livewires who improve on bedtime and most wake-ups but hold on to one stubborn waking until you're about ready to throw in the towel, and then on Day Twelve, they finally sleep all the way through the night.

Chapter twelve discusses how to know if you're moving forward. Try to trust the process for a while. It takes time and grit to get to the goal line.

Days Seven to Nine: Position Three

BEDTIME: MOVE YOUR CHAIR TO THE DOOR (BUT STILL INSIDE THE ROOM)

In this position, you are going to be doing exactly what you've been doing since Day Four—just from farther away. For little ones in cribs, this usually isn't too hard. For toddlers and little ones in beds, it can get tricky. Don't worry. In chapters ten and eleven, we give you lots of information on navigating the transition out of the room.

NIGHTTIME WAKE-UPS: DO THE SAME THING YOU DID AT BEDTIME

For any waking (or any nonfeed waking, for babies who are still getting fed), quickly go to the crib / bed to check to make sure all is well, and then return to the chair and stay until they're back asleep.

ARE WE THERE YET? TRACKING PROGRESS

By this time, you could be seeing bits of improvement in the time it takes your livewire to fall sleep and/or in the spans between wake-ups and/or in their ability to go back to sleep after a waking without your help. The wins may not be the same each night, but you should be seeing them. Don't worry if improvement happens in fits and starts. That's normal. It can take a while for livewires to really get their sleep ducks in a row.

If you have gotten this far and it's still awful / bumpy, or if there was some progress that has now completely stalled, check chapter twelve to see if there's something getting in the way.

Days Ten to Twelve: Position Four

BEDTIME: MOVE THE CHAIR OUTSIDE THE DOOR BUT IN VIEW

Here, you're making another small move, this time outside the door, but where your livewire can still see you. For little ones under two, moving away is usually not a big deal. For separation-sensitive toddlers, this can be where they get a little worried. This doesn't mean you change your strategy. Consistency and reassurance are still the name of the game for toddlers in cribs and beds. (More on this in chapter eleven.)

NIGHTTIME WAKE-UPS: DO THE SAME THING YOU DID AT BEDTIME

For any waking (or nonfeed waking, for babies who are still getting fed), quickly go to the crib / bed to check to make sure all is well, then return to the chair and stay until they're back asleep.

COMMON WHAT IFS AT THIS POSITION

"What if having the door open lets in too much light from the hallway?"

This is a common challenge. I've had parents put a blanket in the open doorway or leave the door open only a crack so they can still be heard through it. I've also seen parents close the door and use the monitor to speak to the child in the room. You may have to improvise a little.

Days Thirteen to Fifteen: Position Five

BEDTIME AND WAKE-UPS AT NIGHT: MOVE THE CHAIR OUTSIDE THE DOOR BUT OUT OF VIEW

For this position, close the door except for a crack and sit where your child can't see you but can still hear you, like around the corner of the doorway. Check chapters ten and eleven for more about navigating this transition.

Day Sixteen On: Position Six

BEDTIME AND NIGHTTIME WAKINGS: PERIODIC CHECK-INS

Hopefully, by now, sleep is almost completely handled. Starting with Day Sixteen, you will be periodically checking in with your child until they fall asleep. You can decide how frequently these check-ins happen. You could do them at set time intervals (for example, every five minutes) or as needed. Just go to the door (unless they're really crying and you think something is up, of course; then you can go in) and shush a bit. We'll talk about a few more details for older livewires who get a little antsy about your being out of sight in chapter eleven.

WHERE IS THE FINISH LINE (OR, HOW TO KNOW WHEN YOU'RE "DONE")?

We've talked a lot about how to navigate concerns that the process isn't working or how to detect progress . . . but what does "done" look like?

Here's the great news: YOU get to decide that. What's "good enough" for you? Maybe you get to the point where your three- or four-year-old is going to bed without drama, sleeping in their own bed until 2 AM, and then comes silently into your room and goes to sleep on their floor bed—and that feels okay . . . at least for now. If you want your eleven-month-old to sleep in the crib all night without a feed, that's awesome. *You* get to decide what good sleep looks like in your house.

Wherever your goal line is: Once you arrive there, please give yourself and your child a big pat on the back.

The next two chapters will give you more specifics about the previous steps based on your livewire's age and sleep location. (You can use these to add notes to your Change the Pattern Worksheet.) Chapter ten covers livewires roughly three years and younger (mostly in cribs). Chapter eleven covers livewires roughly three years and up (mostly in beds). Please feel free to use whatever strategies fit your livewire's developmental level and sleep location.

We're also going to cover, for each age group, how to stay on course. We'll point out where the traps are so that you can avoid them. Most important, we're going to give you the confidence to keep moving forward even when it looks a little chaotic. Livewires take their time getting on board when things change. We have to trust that they can learn a new way.

OUR TRIP CHECKLIST

- ☑ You know you are on a different path.
- ☑ You understand your livewire's temperament strengths and challenges.
- ☑ You understand the link between temperament and sleep issues.
- ☑ Your child is ready:
    - ☑ Over six months
    - ☑ No upcoming disruptions
    - ☑ No physiological issues that affect sleep
- ☑ You are ready (or as ready as you can be).
- ☑ You understand the Big Four sources of sleep issues.
- ☑ Big Strategy #1: You know how to avoid that second wind.
- ☑ Big Strategy #2: You have a solid, consistent bedtime routine.
- ☑ Big Strategy #3 and #4: You know how to change the go-to-sleep and back-to-sleep patterns and are prepared to be more consistent than you've ever been before.
- ☐ You know how to track progress.
- ☐ You know how to diagnose and fix any problems that arise.
- ☐ BETTER SLEEP!

CHAPTER 10

Ins and Outs for Six Months up to Three Years (Mostly in Cribs)

> ❰❰ If you have flipped to this chapter without having read chapter nine, please go back and do that. This chapter will not be helpful if you haven't read the previous one.

The last chapter outlined the key elements of the Shuffle. While the main ideas are the same regardless of age, there *are* some extra ins and outs based on age and sleep location that are going to be critical to know.

In this chapter, we are generally talking about babies and toddlers in cribs in their own rooms. However, we know that some parents of younger livewires are using floor beds or have moved their toddlers into a big kid bed. Or the crib is still in your room. We will absolutely offer modifications for these. For folks who are going to continue safely co-sleeping, that's totally fine, but we encourage you to consider working on go-to-sleep skills in the crib for those first few hours of the evening. A mobile baby alone on a big bed is not safe. Getting them to sleep in a crib for at least the first part of the night gives them some independent go-to-sleep skills and means you don't have to go to bed when they do (and you might just get a few hours to be a grown-up).

We're going to talk about working on *both* bedtime and through the night, but remember, you can absolutely go slower or work on only part of the night if you want. The secret sauce is going to be gradually moving toward doing less and being consistent with what you've chosen to tackle—whatever that happens to be.

Days One to Three: Position One (Beside the Crib / Bed)

Overview for Livewires in Cribs
BEDTIME

- Make sure that a feed is not the last thing that happens before they go into the crib.
- Get them into the crib, ready for sleep but awake.
- Sit in a chair *right beside the crib*, patting / shushing / humming intermittently.
- If they get really upset, you can pick them up to calm them, but put them back down once they're calm and keep going.
- Stay until they're completely asleep.

WAKE-UPS

- For babies a year or so and under, you will decide whether any feeds are going to happen and when (see page 206 for how to do this).
  - When it's time for a feed, get to them quickly, feed them, and get them back into the crib. (You don't have to put them back into bed awake.)
  - For *all other* wakings, coach them back to sleep by doing exactly what you did at bedtime (sit right beside the crib, pat / shush / hum intermittently).

- For babies / toddlers over a year, coach them back to sleep by doing exactly what you did at bedtime (sit right beside the crib, pat / shush / hum intermittently).
- If they get really upset, you can pick them up to calm them, but put them back down once they're calm and keep going.
- Stay until they're completely asleep.

Overview for Livewires (Under Three) in Floor Beds or Toddler Beds

BEDTIME

- Make sure that a feed is not the last thing that happens before they go to bed.
- Get them in bed, ready for sleep but awake.
- Sit beside the bed intermittently patting / shushing / humming.
- If they get really upset, you can pick them up or hug them to calm them, but once they're calm, encourage them to lie back down. Keep going.
- Stay until they are completely asleep.

WAKE-UPS

- For babies a year (or so) and under, decide when feeds happen (page 207).
  - When it's time for a feed, get to them quickly, feed them, and get them back into bed. (They do not have to be awake.)
  - For *all other* wakings, coach them back to sleep exactly how you did at bedtime.
- For babies / toddlers over a year, coach them back to sleep by doing exactly what you did at bedtime.
- If they are old enough to come out of their room to find you and you haven't installed a baby gate, first walk them silently back to their room, then resume your bedtime position and pat / shush / hum intermittently until they're completely asleep.

- If they get really upset, you can pick up or hug them to calm them, but once they're calm, encourage them to lie back down. Keep going.
- Stay until they are completely asleep.

Overview for Livewires Who Are Co-sleeping (After Bedtime in a Crib)

BEDTIME

- Follow the guidelines for babies / toddlers in cribs.

WAKE-UPS

- For babies a year or so and under, you will decide when feeds happen (page 206).
  - When it's time for a feed, do it quickly, and get them back to sleep.
  - For *all other* wakings, coach them back to sleep in the bed with intermittent patting / shushing / humming until they're completely asleep.
- For babies / toddlers over a year, coach them back to sleep with intermittent patting / shushing / humming until they're completely asleep.

BEDTIME: WHAT TO DO AND HOW TO AVOID CURVEBALLS

Remember, bedtime is the *most important* moment for teaching new sleep skills. This is when we establish a new template for how your livewire can go to sleep (and later, back to sleep) without physical help from you.

The big change on this first night is that you're going to be getting your livewire into the crib (or bed) with less (or none) of whatever you've been doing so far (bouncing on a ball, rocking, feeding, lying with them). If you need to take a couple of days first to wean down the circus of things you're doing now, that's fine. Slow down the yoga ball bouncing, move the feed gradually further away from being put down—whatever you have to do in preparation. Once you're ready, start on the Day One plan.

We're going to ditch the word drowsy and put them down awake.

We know you've been told to put your little one in the crib "drowsy but awake," and you may think you've been doing that because their eyes are a little open when you go to transfer them. This is not what we're shooting for here. When adults think of "drowsy," we think "eyelids starting to droop, maybe nodding off" because that's what *we* look like when we're drowsy. For a baby, those behaviors signal they are already pretty far down the road to sleep, and they're only having to go a little of the way to sleep on their own. When they wake up at night, they'll need your help to get back to that level of drowsy again.

If it's only taking your child five minutes to fall asleep, you may think, *Yay! At least bedtime is really easy!* Then you're puzzled about why they can't fall back asleep as easily in the middle of the night. Falling asleep in five minutes means that whatever you were doing during the bedtime routine or right before putting them down got them 80 percent of the way to sleep, and they really only went 20 percent on their own. If they wake up at night and are 50 percent awake, they'll need your help to get back to 80 percent before they can take it from there.

We want your livewire to learn how to go virtually *all* the way from awake to asleep so that, when they wake up at night, they'll know how to get back to sleep on their own. Instead of putting them down "drowsy but awake," we really want to put them down *ready for sleep* (fed, dry, loved) *but awake*. Good timing and an effective, predictable routine should be enough to get them there.

We can expect that they will lose it.

I know it feels daunting. I know you're thinking, *Are you serious? This live-wire is used to a full-court press of strategies to just get them to fall asleep at all. I'm supposed to just put them in the crib? Are you nuts?* I know. Really, I do. Here's the thing:

**There's no move you can make that's
so small they won't notice.**

You know this is true. Even if you wanted to start super slowly by getting them in bed 99 percent drowsy, the minute you laid them down not 100 percent asleep, their eyes would pop back open as if you just laid them down totally awake. You might as well just go for it. There's honestly nothing that's going to fly under their radar.

You can always calm them down.

At any point in this process that you think your livewire is getting to their upper limit of "okay," you get to pick them up to calm them down. Once they're calm, put them back and keep going . . . even if they just start freaking out again. That's okay. It's important, however, that when you pick them up, you don't just go sit on the yoga ball or hold them the way you used to when putting them to sleep. That's a tease. They're going to think, *Finally! All this nonsense is done. We're going to go back to the old way. Yay!* And when you put them back down, they're going to be shocked and mad. So, pick them up but do something different than you did before. If you used to walk them around, instead stand and bounce a little or sway. We just want to help them calm down. We're not trying to make them drowsy. For kiddos in beds, you can do a good deep-pressure hug instead of a pick-up to help them calm down.

"How do I know when I should pick them up?"

There's no rule about when you can or should pick them up. You don't have to time yourself. You can use your internal alarm system to figure out when they need help. You can pick them up as many times as you need to.

Make sure you pay attention to what *they* do when you pick them up, however. If they immediately fall asleep on your shoulder, it means that they were freaking out to get back to being on you. It was a strategy (bless their hearts), and because you're such an awesome parent, it worked. Next time, just wait a beat or two longer before picking them up to see if you can make them work a teeny bit harder.

Also, over the coming days, be more and more judicious about how much you pick up to calm. With livewires, this can be tricky to figure out. There's a fine line between picking them up when they really need it and picking them up too quickly. There may be some trial and error involved. Just be careful to reduce how often you pick up to calm over time.

"What if they get so upset that they throw up?"

There are some livewires who, in past sleep training attempts, have gotten so worked up that they threw up. And this *can* happen, very occasionally, even in more gradual sleep coaching. But it's rare. Both of us have worked with livewires who had a history of throwing up when parents attempted a Ferber-like approach, but when the parents used the Shuffle, it didn't happen anymore.

If you're really worried that your child might barf, try splitting up their bedtime feed / milk and giving half early in the routine and half nearer to bedtime, rather than all of it nearer to bedtime. During coaching, you can also pick up to calm sooner.

In this process, you get to be supportive and present . . . but you cannot let the intensity of their reaction make you stop in these first couple of nights.

If they do throw up (which, again, is rare), clean everything up, maybe offer a little water, and stay with them until they're asleep. There's no need to start the routine over or do anything more than you were doing already.

WHAT TO DO ABOUT A PACIFIER ADDICT

Pacifiers are tricky. Babies under about nine months or so often aren't yet able to locate and replug them themselves, meaning *you* become the paci wrangler. On the other hand, livewires need all the soothing help they can get, and pacifiers can often be a great tool for keeping distress manageable. You really have two choices:

Ditch it. Sometimes it's easier to work on bedtime without the pacifier, so your livewire learns how to fall asleep and go back to sleep without it. If you're already working on new sleep skills, you might as well add that to the list. Make sure this is a clear decision that doesn't wobble. (You can still keep it for naps, if you need to.)

Keep it but put them in charge of it. When your little one is old enough to locate a pacifier near them and put it in their mouth, you can leave this to them. You can start by only putting the pacifier in their hand once they are in their crib. That way, *they* are in charge of replugging it. Once they're getting the hang of replugging, you can just point to the pacifier and let them grab it. Then, try throwing four or five in the crib at bedtime so they are easy to locate without you. (There are even glow-in-the-dark pacifiers available that make locating one even easier.)

If you notice that your little one is throwing the pacifier on purpose to get you to play, return it *one time*—and after that, if they throw it, it stays on the floor until the next wake-up.

Common what ifs at this position

Livewires in cribs: "What if they just sit / stand up when I put them into the crib?"

If your baby is sitting or standing, don't get pulled into a power struggle of trying to make them lie down. If they sit / stand up, help them lie down *once*. After that, either pat the mattress or put your face down at mattress level so they have to get down to see you. Let *them* do the work of getting back down into a sleep position.

If your baby can stand, but can't yet sit back down, you will have to help them until they master that skill. Make practicing this during the day a priority.

Livewires in cribs: "What if I feel like my sitting there is just making them mad?"

This does happen with some livewires. Sometimes the things we do to help them are just annoying to them. Or the fact that you are *right there* but not doing what they want you to do just drives them up a tree. Generally, in the first three days, we still want you to stay beside them. You can try doing less—don't make eye contact, don't pat *and* shush, just do one thing at a time. Or you can move your chair farther away or sit on the floor instead of the chair. But do see if you can stay in the room with them and push through these first three days.

Mobile livewires in beds: "What if, when I move away, they just crawl over to me?"

This is the main challenge of a little one on a bed. Without a crib railing, they can just scooch over to you. You may need some kind of boundary or barrier. You can try buying a body or bolster pillow that you can put between you (a body pillow can also be a substitute cuddle buddy for your livewire). If that's not working, instead of sitting on the bed or floor, you may need to sit in a chair next to the bed. Try to be as boring and unflustered as possible. When your livewire sees that you aren't going to engage, they'll stop—eventually. It may take a day or two of practicing this for them to see that you really aren't going to play along or change your plan. (If the floor bed is really becoming a struggle, it's not the worst idea to go back to the crib until they're a little older.)

WAKE-UPS: HANDLING THE
MIDDLE OF THE NIGHT

The key to this entire process is a consistent response that encourages a more independent go-to-sleep and back-to-sleep pattern. Whatever you are doing at bedtime, you should be also doing in the middle of the night. That said, some babies still need feeds at night. Because we don't want to confuse them, we plan those feeds and we respond right away. Even though some wake-ups are coaching sessions and some are feeds, if there's a structure to that process, there will be logic to it.

Decide what to do about night feeds.

The nagging worry about hunger is a leading cause of so many failed sleep training attempts. Parents work and work trying to get their crying baby back to sleep, and then end up feeding their baby because the thought that they're just torturing a hungry child won't leave them alone.

Night feeds are not, in themselves, a bad thing. However, we're going to be thoughtful about them so that you can move toward better sleep while feeling confident your child is not starving. Always talk with your pediatrician to get a sense of whether your child needs to feed at night for their development and growth.

Night feeds for infants are up to you.

For babies six to nine months (or even up to almost a year), night feeds are okay and *up to you*. However, we want to plan them ahead of time so that you are stretching your child's ability to go longer between feeds and helping them practice their back-to-sleep skills. We really want you to feel confident and clear about when feeds happen and when they don't. Here's another upside to limiting nighttime feeding: If your livewire wakes *a lot* and gets fed every time, they are consuming a significant number of their calories at night, which can make them less hungry during the day and more likely to wake up hungry again at night. Limiting feeding at night encourages better daytime feeding and therefore better nighttime sleep.

Start by deciding when you think your baby *really* needs to feed. I'm going to encourage you to be bold. Waking is not always caused by hunger. Some happen simply because your child has come into a light stage of sleep and needs to re-engage their go-to-sleep pattern, and that pattern includes feeding. Feeding is how they know to get back to sleep. If your livewire is currently feeding three or four (or more) times at night, they can likely do less than that.

For infants six to eight or nine months, two feeds are reasonable (and definitely better than four!). One way to structure these is to schedule a dream feed (where you wake your baby to feed them, rather than them waking you) right before you go to bed. Then shoot for a four- to six-hour window until the second feed. A schedule like this lets you get a solid stretch of sleep. I've worked with a lot of parents who feed at 10 PM, 1 AM, and 4 AM, and in this scenario, they never get more than a three-hour block of sleep.

If you absolutely can't stretch or you're currently feeding at every wake-up, pick an amount of time you know you can stick with (*"I know my baby can go four hours without a feed, so we'll feed at the first wake-up after 10 PM, 2 AM, and 6 AM"*). Over time, we're going to try to stretch the time between feeds and set our sights on eventually getting you a good chunk of sleep (doesn't that sound amazing?). Then, by nine months or so, you could drop to one feed. It's up to you which of the two you phase out. You could do a dream feed and then have no feeds until morning. Alternatively, you could eliminate the dream feed and only feed after 3 or 4 AM.

It's important to note that dream feeds don't always work for livewires because once they're a little awake, they're *awake*. Only do a dream feed if you know you can get your baby back in the crib easily. If you find that a dream feed means that you're spending an hour getting your livewire back down after you woke them to feed, or they don't really eat much, don't do it. Instead, you could do a set time for this feed—the first wake-up after 10 PM, for example. At all other wake-ups, you'll coach your infant back to sleep the same way you do at bedtime.

Once you decide whether and when you will schedule any feeds, set those feed times clearly (*"We're going to do a dream feed before we go to bed, then no feeds until the first wake-up after 3 AM"*). If it's after 3 AM, you will go to them quickly, feed them, and get them back to sleep. If they fall asleep during the feed, that's okay. Just be sure to do your absolute best to stick to the timing that you have preset. If you decided that you'll feed at the first wake-up after 4 AM, don't let that start sliding to 3 AM, then 2:30, etc. These limits need to be times you can absolutely stick to.

"What if our feed time is 4 AM, and they wake at 3 AM and we're still coaching them to sleep an hour later? Should we just feed them?" This seem logical, for sure. But remember, you don't want to work hard at coaching for an hour and then just feed them because then your child thinks, *Aha! When I wake up, feeding / nursing is an option.* The next time you try to coach them, they may protest *at least* an hour, if not longer. Get them back to sleep first, and then feed them at the *next* wake-up—even if that's only fifteen minutes later.

**We want to avoid capping a bunch of sleep
coaching effort and work with a feed.**

That's why we phrase the feed time as "the first wake-up *after* 4 AM." At each wake-up, it's *either* a feeding session *or* a coaching session, never both.

WORKBOOK TO DO

Write down your schedule for feed(s) on your Change the Pattern Worksheet in the Workbook.

Night feeds for toddlers (over a year)? It's time to ditch those.

If your livewire is older than a year, healthy and growing well, and still nursing or having bottles or cups of milk at night, it's time for those to go. Full stop. Remember, dentists strongly encourage that for children with teeth, every milk feed should be followed by toothbrushing because milk sugar on teeth can cause cavities even at this early age.[63] Also, the possibility of a feed can almost act as an incentive to wake up at night. Those persistent, perceptive livewires can start waking every hour, like they're saying, "Is it time now? How about now?" For healthy children over a year, night feeds are not necessary and are merely a part of their go-to-sleep and back-to-sleep pattern.

You're already going to be changing their usual patterns, so removing nursing or bottles should just be another part of this work. You *can* go cold turkey on these nighttime feedings, but you don't have to. You can wean these feeds by cutting down the number of ounces you offer or minutes that you nurse over three nights (yes, just three) at the same time that you start coaching. Avoid offering water instead. Toddlers aren't thirsty. They're mostly using sucking to help them go to sleep. Offering water won't really move the process forward and can also contribute to soggier diapers that need to be changed during the night. If you really feel like the they might need water at night (because of an illness or your local weather), you can put a spill-proof sippy cup with a small amount of water (no refills) in their crib or by the bed, so they can get it themselves as needed.

How to handle night feeds when you're co-sleeping

It's definitely going to be more challenging to stick to a feed schedule while co-sleeping when your baby knows the source is *right there*. It's also going to be tempting to just nurse your livewire the second they stir because . . . well, it's just easy, and parents of livewires *need* "easy." However, if you're committed to making sleep better, we have to give your child opportunities to practice going back to sleep without nursing every time.

Tips for coaching in the middle of the night while co-sleeping:

- Have your baby sleep next to the non-nursing partner (or, even better, have the nursing partner go into another room and only come in for feeds).
- Have the nursing partner wear a sports bra or zip-up turtleneck so access is not so easy.

What to do if they wake up really early (before 6 AM)

Early rising is a common by-product of messing with a baby or toddler's familiar sleep patterns, and it often starts happening during coaching. If early rising was happening *before* coaching, we have found that it's typically the last piece of the sleep puzzle to resolve. Check chapter 12 for clues as to whether anything besides your work on sleep could be causing the early rising.

Here's how to deal with it in the moment:

Livewires under two: Try to wait until 6 AM to start the day. If they are happily chatting in their crib, it's okay to let them do that until it's time to get up. Little ones under a year who have gone a fair number of hours without a feed may actually be hungry, however. See if offering a quick feed will get them back to sleep for another hour or two. For all other livewires, try to get to them quickly and see if you can coach them back to sleep.

If the clock strikes 6 AM while you're sitting there and it's time to start the day, don't just get them out of the crib and leave the room. Instead, use a little trick that Kim calls a Dramatic Wake-Up: leave the room briefly (count to ten or twenty) and then come back in and turn on the light with a bright, "Good morning! We're getting up!" What this little bit of playacting does is send the message that *you* have decided to start the day, and that decision is not connected to them staying awake (though it totally is). The key here is that we don't want you to coach for a while and then "call it" and just pick them up. That links the two events and gives them a reason to hold out the next time they wake early.

Little ones two and up: Try a wake-up clock. A wake-up clock that turns on or changes color when it's time for the day to start can reinforce to older toddlers that it's still time to stay in bed. Set it for a minimum of 6 AM (if you have an early riser), and when they wake before that time, tell them, "The clock is still red. It's still time for sleeping," and go to your chair. You can also use a Dramatic Wake-Up. Both strategies disconnect "not going back to sleep" from "getting to leave the crib / bed."

Make sure to write your plan for early rising into your Change the Pattern Worksheet.

The challenges of a livewire under three years old in a bed

The biggest downside to having a mobile child under three in some kind of bed is that they can just *leave*. Remember, before they're three years old, a child can *know* what they're supposed to do, but they don't yet have the capacity to use that information to direct their body or control their impulses. This means that you are going to have to (1) install a baby gate or door strap to keep them from roaming the house, (2) babyproof the heck out of their room, and (3) silently walk them back to bed potentially a million times.

> **If your livewire sleeps on a floor bed at night without you, we strongly encourage a baby gate or door strap. You really don't want a young livewire roaming the house.**

In any case, you're going to be doing a lot of taking them back to their bed when they get out of it. Walk them back silently, point out that their wake-up light hasn't turned on yet (if you're using one), and let them get back into bed themselves. Then go sit wherever you were at bedtime. Stay until they're completely asleep. If your child is old enough (at least two and a half or three), make sure you remind them at bedtime about what will happen at nighttime wake-ups.

If this feels like a struggle or like it's not working:

- Do you need to take on a smaller part of the night for right now? (For example, coach only at bedtime, then have someone sleep in your livewire's room for the rest of the night.)
- If you still have the crib set up, can you leave it up, just in case? Or if you've taken it down, can you put it back up? It's not a bad thing to go back to using the crib until they're more ready for a big kid bed.

Expecting your livewire to stay in their bed without getting out at this age may be more than they're developmentally able to handle. You may also have to lower the bar for what can be achieved. You may not get all of what you're hoping for *just yet*, but at least we're working toward getting you *some* of it.

Days Four to Six: Position Two
(Away from the Crib / Bed)

Overview for Livewires in Cribs
BEDTIME

- Continue the same bedtime routine, getting them into the crib ready for sleep but awake.
- Move your chair *a few feet away from the crib* and use only your voice to soothe.
- Expect a bump up in protest on the first day of the move. This is normal.
- If they get really upset, you can pick them up to calm them but put them back down once they're calm and keep going.
- Stay until they are completely asleep.

WAKE-UPS

- If it's time for a predetermined feed (if you're doing them), get to them quickly, feed them, and get them back to sleep.
- Any other time your child wakes, do a quick cribside check and return to the chair until your livewire is asleep again. (If the crib is in your room, do the cribside check and return to your bed and soothe vocally from there.)
- If they get really upset, you can pick them up to calm them but put them back down once they're calm and keep going.
- Stay until they're completely asleep.

Overview for Livewires in Floor Beds or Toddler Beds
BEDTIME

- Continue the same bedtime routine, getting them into bed ready for sleep but awake.
- Move a little away from the bed.
- Use only your voice to calm.

- Expect a bump up in protest on the first day of the move. This is normal.
- If they get really upset, you can still pick up or hug them to calm them but put them back down once they're calm and keep going.
- Stay until they're completely asleep.

WAKE-UPS

- If it's time for a predetermined feed (if you're doing them), get to them quickly, feed them, and get them back to sleep.
- Any other time your child wakes, do a quick check and return to where you were at bedtime until your livewire is asleep again.
- If they get really upset, you can still pick up or hug them to calm them but put them back down once they're calm and keep going.
- Stay until they're completely asleep.

Overview for Livewires Who Are Co-sleeping (After Bedtime in a Crib)
WAKE-UPS

- If you are still doing night feeds, stick to your planned feed windows.
- Make a decisive reduction in whatever you are doing to get your livewire back to sleep and stick to it.

BEDTIME: WHAT TO DO AND HOW
TO AVOID CURVEBALLS

Day Four is when you make your first move. For livewires in cribs, this means moving your chair a few feet away from the crib or about half-way between the crib and the doorway. If the room is small and your first move is practically to the door, that's okay. You can skip Position Three (page 218). The key is to *move*.

Day Four might be bumpy.

Hopefully, you saw *something* shift in the first three days. If you did, good job, you. (If not, see chapter twelve.) However, don't be surprised if protest on Day Four ticks up again. Day Four is the first move away, which can throw your perceptive livewire ("*Wait. What's happening now?*"), and this is a normal response to change. On the fourth day, your child will typically make one more push for things to go back to the way they were. If you can tough it out, the resistance should mellow out on Day Five and beyond. Don't let Day Four's extra dose of pushback make you think you're off course. You're not. This is temporary.

Remember: "Away" is away.

Day Four needs to be a decisive move. When you make this first move and you are "away from the crib / bed," for example, the only touching that should happen is pick up to calm. Resist the impulse to go back to the side of the crib to do one more pat or help them lie down. Going back to crib / bedside is going to make this move mushy. You need to signal your confidence that they can tolerate you not being right there beside them.

You can still pick up or hug to calm.

Hopefully, on Day Five, after the bump up on Day Four, the protest is mellowing out. But if there are moments of more intense freak-out, you can still always pick up to calm. This is a critical piece for our intense, persistent livewires. We really don't want them to work themselves up to a point where they are beyond the ability to downshift. The *only* time to question whether you should have picked them up is when they fall asleep on you as soon as you do. In that instance, consider waiting just a hair longer before picking them up the next time. And do your best to reduce using this strategy over time if you can.

Common what ifs at this position

Livewires in cribs: "What if I still feel like my presence is making it worse?"

If you have reached Position Two and you still feel like shushing (or whatever your calming method is) is making it worse, the most sensitive thing you can do is give your livewire some space and see if that helps them hunker down. First, try not offering eye contact, or only do one sensory modality at a time (eye contact *or* shushing). Or maybe humming or white noise is better, or try silence. You can also try moving to a spot where they can't see you, but you're still present in the room.

Livewires in cribs in their parents' room: "What if the minute they wake up and see me, it's 'game on'?"

For some very engaged livewires, seeing you right over there in your bed is all they need to think, *Oh right! Mom and Dad!* and then wake up more fully. In these situations, it's a good idea to have a visual barrier between the crib and your bed. A room screen or other strategy that obscures or blocks their view of you can approximate them having their own space.

Livewires in beds: "What if they won't stay put at bedtime?"

The trick now is going to be moving away without your little one just getting up and coming over to you. If they get up, you can go over and pat the mattress to see if they will get back in bed. If they insist on lying on the floor or somewhere else, maybe that's okay for now. We don't want you getting in a power struggle over them lying on the bed.

If your mobile baby or toddler keeps climbing into your lap or playing around and it's truly becoming a struggle, you may need to go more slowly. Try backing up a step: Start with a full cuddle, and then, after one or two nights, move a few inches away but intermittently put a hand on them, then move a few more inches away, etc.

If going more slowly doesn't work, it's not the end of the world if you need to pivot back to coaching them in a crib for bedtime and then co-sleeping on the floor bed for the rest of the night. Even if your livewire is a world-class climber, there are ways to keep a kiddo in the crib. See page 135 for these hacks.

WAKE-UPS: HANDLING THE MIDDLE OF THE NIGHT

For any nonfeed wake-up, after a quick crib- or bedside check-in, you will go to the chair again and periodically shush until they're back asleep.

Common what ifs at this position

Livewires in beds: "What if they just keep getting out of their bed whenever they wake up?"

Hopefully, you've installed a baby gate or door strap, and so when they wake up at night, they will be calling you from there. If you don't have a gate (or they've climbed it . . . yikes) and they suddenly appear in your room (or your bed), remember that you will need to walk them silently back to their room. In both scenarios, remind them that they're supposed to stay in bed until their wake-up clock turns on / changes color. Then, sit in your chair until they're asleep again.

Livewires who co-sleep: "What if I'm right next to them at night? How do I 'move away'?"

It's true—when you're co-sleeping, you can't really move away. But moving away physically is just one way of reducing how much a parent is participating in the go-to-sleep and back-to-sleep process. In a co-sleeping context, you will be working on reducing what you are doing in response to nonfeed wake-ups. You could have the baby sleep on the non-nursing partner's side. You could gradually move away by lying on your back, then rolling to your other side. You can taper down your vocal support by speaking more softly or waiting longer intervals between shushes. Tapering down is harder when co-sleeping, but it can be done.

Days Seven to Nine: Position Three (At the Door)

Overview for Livewires in Cribs
BEDTIME AND WAKE-UPS

- Move your chair *to the door*, still using only your voice to calm.
- If they get really upset, you can pick up or hug to calm (sparingly).
- Stay until they're completely asleep.
- For any waking that's not a feed, do exactly what you did at bedtime. (If the crib is in your room, do the cribside check and return to your bed and soothe vocally from there.)

Overview for Livewires in Floor Beds or Toddler Beds
BEDTIME AND WAKE-UPS

- Make another move away (physically or, if co-sleeping, by reducing your vocal soothing).
- For any waking that's not a feed, do exactly what you did at bedtime.
- If they get really upset, you can hug to calm (sparingly).

Overview for Livewires Who Are Co-sleeping (After Bedtime in a Crib)
WAKE-UPS

- Stick to your limits for any night feeds.
- Reduce your interaction / soothing even more.

BEDTIME AND WAKE-UPS: AVOIDING CURVEBALLS AND HANDLING THE MIDDLE OF THE NIGHT

By this time, you should feel like you're really getting the hang of this and you are just repeating the same steps in new positions.

For livewires under two in a crib, there doesn't appear to be a big difference between their parent being *a little* away from the crib and *more* away. For these little ones, the biggest lift is in the first four or five days. For toddlers, it can get tricky as you start moving toward the door, but as long as you're prepared for it, you can navigate those rough waters. Keep reading.

For many if not most livewires, those new sleep skills should really be kicking in by this point. If there are still some stubborn spots (a waking that's still happening, early morning rising), don't despair. Sometimes you have to really keep at it to make these new patterns truly fall into place (especially the early rising). Just keep consistently moving forward. If you are still struggling or there hasn't been huge improvement, however, check chapter twelve for help figuring out why.

Common what ifs at this position

Livewires in the parents' room: "What if I'm right there in my bed? How do I move to Position Three during wake-ups?"

When you are sleeping in the same room as your livewire, moving away in the middle of the night is not always possible because you're going to be in the same spot you've been in this whole time: your bed.

Here, as when co-sleeping, moving away is really about reducing your participation in your livewire's go-to-sleep and back-to-sleep pattern. When you can't reduce *physical* presence, you will focus on reducing your *vocal* presence. You can reduce the volume of your shushing or pause longer between shushes. It almost doesn't matter what you choose to change as long as you are gradually doing less and stretching their ability to get back to sleep without as much help from you.

Livewires in beds: "What if my toddler isn't letting me be outside the room?"

Moving farther away for some livewires in a bed is no big deal. For others, it's a very big deal. Getting them to stay in their bed without you can be a big challenge when they're under three years. Try to stay the course, but if you really hit a roadblock, and you can't move them back to a crib, you may need to reduce your expectations until they are a little older and have developed more self-regulation and impulse control. Maybe just focus on achieving a better bedtime or easier wake-ups for now.

Days Ten to Twelve: Position Four (Outside the Door but in View)

Overview for Livewires in Cribs, Floor Beds, or Toddler Beds
BEDTIME AND WAKE-UPS

- Move your chair *out into the hallway but still in view*.
- If they get really upset, you can pick up or hug to calm (very sparingly).
- Stay until they're completely asleep.
- For any waking that's not a feed, do exactly what you did at bedtime.

Overview for Livewires Who Are Co-sleeping (after Bedtime in a Crib)
WAKE-UPS

- Reduce your interaction even more.

BEDTIME AND WAKE-UPS: AVOIDING CURVEBALLS AND HANDLING THE MIDDLE OF THE NIGHT

For little ones younger than two or so, moving outside the room often isn't a big deal. However, livewires two and up (who are at the height of true separation anxiety) start to get nervous when you move to being outside the room. They may have been fine while you were *in* the room but now have a real issue with you looking like you're leaving. (Of course, you're *not* leaving.) They may start lobbying (yelling, insisting, demanding) to get you to come back inside. Know that this may happen and be ready for it. It's a little bit like Day One again: You are going to have to allow them to express their displeasure with what's happening *and* keep going.

Common what ifs at this position

Two-year-old livewires in a crib: "What if my livewire freaks out about my being outside the door?"

For two-year-olds, who are developmentally experiencing some separation anxiety, it makes sense that this step isn't easy for them. Still, because you are going to be right there in the hallway until they're asleep and you will help calm them down if they need it, you can push through, knowing that on the second or third day of this position, they'll catch on.

If they do continue to really freak out after a day or two, the solution is *not* to go back to staying in the room. (*Don't* do it. You will get stuck.) Instead, try breaking this move into smaller steps over a few days. Start in the doorway and make micromoves every night or two. As long as you stay supportive and consistent, your livewire can gradually learn to tolerate your being farther away.

Two-year-old livewires in a bed: "What if my livewire comes to the door / gate and begs me to come back into the room?"

If livewires over two in *cribs* get nervous, little ones in a *bed* can really get jumpy. Toddlers might get up and go to the door to try to get you to come back inside the room; this is where having a baby gate will really help. Reassure them that you will stay right there until they're asleep. Explain to them that they are the boss of their sleep and that it's their job to learn how to get there. They might ultimately fall asleep on the other side of the gate a few feet from you. That's okay. You can pick them up and move them to the bed once they're asleep. This behavior shouldn't last forever, and you can absolutely call it a win for now—they still fell asleep with less of *you* involved.

If it's *really* difficult for them, you can break this move into microsteps, similar to what we suggested for those over two in cribs. Instead of going straight from at the door to outside the door (the other side of the gate), maybe you move an inch a night, so you are gradually scaffolding their tolerance for you being out of the room. Remember, it's okay to go slower—*as long as* you keep moving.

Days Thirteen to Fifteen: Position Five (Outside the Door and Out of View)

Overview for Livewires in Cribs, Floor Beds, or Toddler Beds
BEDTIME AND WAKE-UPS

- Move your chair *out into the hallway out of view*. This could be just around the corner of the door. They should be able to hear you but not see you.
- For any waking that's not a feed, do exactly what you did at bedtime.
- If they get really upset, you can pick up or hug to calm (very sparingly) and reassure them that you're in the hallway.
- Stay until they're completely asleep.

Overview for Babies / Toddlers Who Are Co-sleeping (after Bedtime in a Crib)
WAKE-UPS

- Stick to your limits for any night feeds.
- Continue reducing interaction.

BEDTIME AND WAKE-UPS: AVOIDING CURVEBALLS AND HANDLING THE MIDDLE OF THE NIGHT

Livewires under two(ish) are hopefully really hitting their stride. With younger ones, it typically gets easier over time. With toddlers it can get a little harder because they feel your absence more keenly. Remember—*keep going.* If you don't want to be stuck forever in their room while they fall asleep, you have to persist in helping them get better at tolerating not being able to see you at bedtime and wake-ups. Believe it or not, some practice with separation is a good thing. Make sure you are still occasionally shushing to reassure and let them know that you're still there even though they can't see you.

Day Sixteen and Beyond: Position Six (Periodic Check-Ins)

Overview for Livewires in Cribs, Floor Beds, or Toddler Beds
BEDTIME AND WAKE-UPS

- After you get them in bed at bedtime, leave the room and come back only for periodic check-ins from the door.
- For wake-ups, do a brief cribside check to make sure everything is okay, then leave the room, checking in periodically until they're asleep.

Overview for Babies / Toddlers Who Are Co-sleeping (after Bedtime in a Crib)
WAKE-UPS

- Do a brief check and go back to sleep.

BEDTIME AND WAKE-UPS: AVOIDING CURVEBALLS AND HANDLING THE MIDDLE OF THE NIGHT

Here, you will be just briefly checking in periodically from the doorway, though we hope that, by now, there's little to do. In many cases, by this stage, sleep is pretty good—even for livewires. If you have any stubborn remaining challenges or you are stuck in an earlier position, chapter twelve will help you figure out where you veered off the path.

┌───┐
WORKBOOK TO DO

Make sure you add your notes from this chapter to your Sleep Plan Worksheet. Then, use all the notes you've made to fill out the Sleep Plan Road Map, which will be your guide for navigating this new process.
└───┘

Let's Talk About Improving Naps (Finally!)

So far, we haven't really said anything about naps except "make sure you get enough of them in any way you can." You really don't want to be trying to sleep coach an overtired livewire who just struggled all day trying to learn to nap independently. In general, we *strongly* recommend waiting to do nap coaching until *after* nighttime is in place. Nap coaching by itself can be a lot of work, and doing both at the same time is usually way too much.

It is possible that once nighttime skills kick in, naps will get easier and/ or better. We've seen it happen. I've also seen situations where even though parents get their livewire to sleep great at night, no amount of nap coaching made a dent in daytime behaviors. Some parents, once nighttime sleep is handled, decide to just let naps be what they are (as long as their livewire is getting *some* sleep during the day).

HOW TO WORK ON INDEPENDENT NAPS

If you *are* ready to work on coaching your livewire to nap independently in the crib, here are the basic steps. These are almost identical to what you will have done for bedtime. You'll just be applying those same skills to naps.

1. **Double check your livewire's nap targets.** Make sure you know how much naptime you're shooting for. Check page 115 for targets by age.
2. **Have a brief nap routine.** Give your livewire some transition time (lower the lights, read a quiet book) ahead of when their wake window ends and then do a very shortened version of their nighttime routine. If your livewire naps well at daycare, but not at home, find out what they do to prepare for the nap. Is there a song they play? Try to mimic what happens there.
3. **Follow the same sequence of steps you followed at bedtime.** For nap coaching, you will start back at Position One. However, instead of keeping at it as long as it takes for your child to fall asleep, you will need to put a limit on how long you try to get them to nap. Otherwise, one nap bumps right up into the next one. An hour is what we usually suggest, but if that's too big an ask, choose an amount of time that you know you can stick to (*"I'll try for forty minutes"*).
4. **Use a Dramatic Wake-Up.** If they don't fall asleep in the window you have set, do a Dramatic Wake-Up: Leave the room, count to ten or twenty, then come in with a bright, "Okay! We're getting

up!" to communicate that *you* are ending the nap attempt, not their delay or pushback.

5. **Don't wait until another wake window goes by.** If they didn't nap at all during that earlier attempt, try for another nap as soon as they seem tired. Even if that's just a half-hour later, try the whole process again.

6. **Have an emergency nap backup plan.** If they are supposed to have multiple naps in a day, and the first one (or two) were terrible or didn't happen, don't try to coach them for their last nap. Just get them to sleep however you can (though avoid holding or feeding to sleep; instead try a ride in the car or stroller, etc.), so that they're not a cranky basket case for bedtime. Make sure you wake them by 5 or 5:30 PM so you can still have a reasonable lights-out time.

7. **If they don't get a good nap, move bedtime earlier.** If your live-wire still doesn't get adequate downtime during the day, be sure to make bedtime a little earlier so you aren't facing a double dose of overtiredness.

HOW TO LENGTHEN NAPS THAT ARE TOO SHORT

If your livewire is able to fall asleep on their own for naps, but then only sleeps thirty or forty minutes at a time, you can use the same strategy to help them learn to sleep longer, too. We really want a nap to be at least forty-five minutes long. If they wake up in less than forty-five minutes, try for another chunk of time (thirty or forty-five minutes) to coach them *back* to sleep. Even if they only go back to sleep for ten more minutes, that's a win. The goal here is to get them to learn how to connect sleep cycles so that they're not waking up completely every time they move into light sleep.

Nap coaching can be a lot of work for the parents of any child. With livewires, oh boy. It can take a few weeks of dedication. As long as you're making progress, keep going, but also follow your gut. If your livewire is sleeping well at night, you might be able to lighten up on your nap work.

If you've really tried with naps and you hit a dead end, this may have to be another "call it good" moment. Continue to get naps whatever way works for you.

IF NAPS AREN'T HAPPENING, TRY QUIET TIME

Taking the time to nap coach your toddler is possible if they're an only child. It's a different story if you also have one or more other children at home. You just can't do the amount of work it could take to get them to sleep. Plus, livewires just get better at fighting naps the older they get. While children under four almost always need an actual nap during the day, it's just not always possible for livewires. In both cases, you may need to pivot to Quiet Time (and an earlier bedtime) for a while.

Quiet Time is a brief bit of quiet, nonstimulating activity that gives your livewire's brain at least a little time to decompress. It doesn't have to be long, and your child doesn't have to actually sleep. Here are some possible Quiet Time strategies for livewire toddlers in cribs:

- Close the blinds or curtains and dim the lights. If possible, turn on special fairy lights or other colored lights that are only used for Quiet Time.
- Have a special pillow or special stuffed animals or activity books that come out only for Quiet Time.
- If they're old enough, have them listen to a recorded sleep visualization story. Listening to a story gives them something to focus on while they're lying down, and it might even help them fall asleep.
- If you must, a quiet video in a darkened room can also work.

Really, *any* rest is better than no rest, and any reduction in stimulation can help them reset a little.

>> If your livewire is close to three, you may want to read on. Otherwise, you can skip to chapter twelve to learn how to track your progress and what to do if things start going off the rails.

CHAPTER 11

Ins and Outs for Three Years and Up (Mostly in Beds)

> ◀◀ If you have flipped to this chapter without having read chapter nine, please go back and do that. This chapter will not be helpful if you haven't read the previous one.

Chapter nine outlined the key elements of the Shuffle. While the main ideas are the same regardless of age, there *are* some extra ins and outs based on age and sleep location that are going to be critical to know.

In this chapter, we are generally talking about livewires older than three in beds in their own rooms. While older livewires generally start in their own room, it can be the middle of the night that's different . . . and maybe that's your issue. As always, you can decide what sleep location or locations work best for your family. If it's okay that your livewire comes quietly into your room in the middle of the night and you all sleep well, that's fine. Feel free to pick and choose what you want to improve.

We're going to talk about working on *both* bedtime and through the night, but remember, you can absolutely go slower or only work on part of the night if you want. The secret sauce is going to be gradually moving toward doing less and being consistent with what you've chosen to tackle— whatever that happens to be.

Days One to Three: Position One (Beside the Bed)

Overview of This Position
BEDTIME

- Review the Bedtime Chart during the day to give your child a heads-up about what's happening that night, including where you'll be sitting.
- Have a good pre-routine routine and a solid, consistent bedtime routine.
- Check items off the chart as you go.
- Get your livewire in bed and sit in a chair *right beside the bed*.
- You can shush / hum / rub their back intermittently, as long as *you* control the touch.
- If they get really upset, use a hug to help calm them. Once they're calm, return to your chair.
- Stay until they're completely asleep.

WAKE-UPS

- If they're supposed to stay in their room, walk them back to their bed, and let them get in the bed themselves.
- If you are using a wake-up clock, point to it and remind them that it's still time for sleep.
- Sit in the chair, and do exactly what you did at bedtime (pat / shush / hum intermittently).
- Stay until they're completely asleep.

THE NEXT DAY

- Remember to review the Bedtime Chart and any progress the next morning.
- Give lots of attention to what went well and ignore what didn't.

BEDTIME: WHAT TO DO AND HOW TO AVOID CURVEBALLS

Remember, bedtime is the *most important* moment for teaching new sleep skills. This is when we establish the template for how your livewire can go to sleep (and later, back to sleep) without physical help from you.

The big change on this first night is that you're going to be getting your livewire into bed with less (or no) physical help. If you need to take a couple of days first to wean down the circus of things you're doing now, that's fine. Offer a tactile substitute for your hand / eyebrow / hair, sit up in the bed, etc.—whatever you have to do in preparation. Once you're ready, start on the Day One plan.

Review and rehearse.

Don't forget to review the chart earlier in the day and rehearse any changes to their routine. Make absolutely sure that you're not springing anything new on your livewire at bedtime. Make sure, too, that you have practiced anything new ahead of time.

Use a wake-up clock and remind them at bedtime.

A wake-up clock that turns on or changes color at whatever time you set can help your livewire know when it's time for sleep and when it's time to wake up. Let them know that they're supposed to stay in their room until the light turns on/changes color and then you will start the day.

When the lights go out, conversation time is over.

If you have a very verbal little one who just seems to build up conversational steam as the lights go out, turning the light off is a great boundary to set between conversation time and sleep time. Livewires are great at coming up with all kinds of last-minute questions, stories, and ideas to delay going to sleep. It's easy to get pulled into it. Try to establish a rule that says once the light goes out, conversation time is done for the day.

Try to be verbally boring.

Once lights are out, if you have to say anything, avoid using a lot of words. Getting into a debate or lots of explanation about why you made a particular decision, reminding them about their chart, or telling them why it is time to go to sleep is an invitation for engagement and/or debate. Don't do it. You've already carefully laid out the bedtime steps and have reminded them. You don't have to do any more explaining.

Have a short list of go-to phrases that you say over and over in response to whatever they throw at you. Instead of saying, "Time for sleep now. Your body needs rest, so get under the covers and close your eyes," just be a boring conversation partner: "Uh-huh. Night-night" or "Mm-hmm . . . night-night." There are no other words but "night-night" (or "time for sleep," "sleepy time," etc.). Once the lights are off, all focus should be on shutting down and going to sleep.

Remember, you control the touch.

With older livewires, it's easy to end up with your hand or other body part being their lovey as they fall asleep. You will really need to control the touch. Don't let them hold your finger or hand. Put your hand on top of theirs so that you can remove it from time to time. You can also redirect their hand to any substitution you've made (stuffed animal, body pillow, etc.; see page 157). Remember, any input that's attached to *you* means you are going to be on call in the middle of the night, every night.

Remember to taper down any physical soothing.

Even across these first few days, do your best to taper off any touching that you're doing so that the move on Day Four isn't such a shock. If you've been rubbing their back, for example, take bigger and bigger breaks between back rubs or slow down how much you're doing. In just a few days, it's going to be done, so do your best to wean it over the first few days.

If they get really upset, use a hug to calm them.

For babies, we pick them up when they get really upset. For kiddos in beds, this might be harder to do as they grow. A good deep-pressure hug can be a great alternative to help them calm down. As soon as they're calmer, return to your original position.

Common What Ifs at This Position

"What if my livewire gets out of bed, climbs on me, throws their toys, or starts to play at bedtime?"

Mobile livewires in a bed can be a three-ring circus. Ideally, you will plan for this inevitability ahead of time. The Bedtime Chart task included some planning for what will happen in the middle of the night if they get out of bed. Plan for what you will do in response to shenanigans. Remember, you don't want to be making decisions or trying to set limits on the fly.

Here are just a few ideas:

Pick your battles. At this point, we're not going to worry about where they fall asleep. Try to avoid a power struggle over having them lie down in bed. If they get out of bed, you can pat the mattress to indicate that you want them to get back in. If they choose to lie on the floor or a beanbag chair or a pile of stuffed animals while you're sitting there, that may have to be okay for this first part of the process. Move them to their bed once they're asleep.

Use a baby gate or door strap. Having some kind of barrier provides the same feeling of containment that a crib used to provide. It also gives you a way to retreat temporarily without closing the door if there are shenanigans; a closed door can really throw a livewire with separation worries. Definitely show them the gate *during the day*, and rehearse what it will be like for them to be in bed with the gate there. You can tell them that the gate is to remind them that they're supposed to stay in bed once the lights are out.

Use the if / when limit setting format. If there are shenanigans (like they keep getting out of bed or they're goofing around), you can say, "If you choose to play / climb / throw toys, I will sit in the hall on the other side of the gate. When you are calm / in bed, I will come back." You may have to do it calmly a few times before they see you mean business.

Be as unflustered and unflappable as you can be. We want your responses to be as boring as possible so that there's no attention payoff for their shenanigans. We know, this can be a huge challenge if you are already at the end of your mother-loving rope. Take lots of deep breaths and know that even if it looks like this process is nowhere near working, it is. You just have to keep at it.

"What if they say they're scared, their tummy hurts, or their blanket is bunchy?"

Livewires are smart enough to know what kinds of requests really get us. It's hard to know when something is a real issue and when it's just strategic. The Bedtime Chart can help front-load some of these requests and prevent problems, but you will have to move forward very carefully with your parenting antennae alerted to whether any new fear / pain / request is just a tactic. The second you realize that "fixing the blanket" is showing signs of becoming a "thing," set a limit: Fix the blanket one time, and after that, that's it. (The next day, practice having them fix the blanket themselves.) If the issue is a fear of the dark or something else, reread pages 152–156 on how to address these tricky fears.

"What if it's taking them a million years to fall asleep?"

That might happen on these first few nights. As they practice over sub-sequent nights, though, the time to fall asleep should improve. Even if it doesn't, that may be okay. Some bright little ones just take a long time to fall asleep. If your livewire is contentedly singing or talking to themselves, that's fine. We can't *make* them go to sleep. What we're working toward is you not having to be there for it.

Keep track in your log of how long it's truly taking them so you'll be able to see whether it's changing. But don't worry too much about it in these first several days. If it continues, we may need to add a strategy or investi-gate further. Try to be patient with it for now.

NIGHTTIME WAKE-UPS: DO THE SAME THING YOU DID AT BEDTIME

You need to be really clear on what the rules are for what happens in the middle of the night because you won't be thinking as clearly. Are they sup-posed to stay in their room all night? If not, what time is okay for them to . . . what? Come into your room and sleep on a floor bed? Co-sleep? It's up to you. Just make sure you're crystal clear on the answer, put it in the chart, and let your livewire know repeatedly what the rules are.

Stick to your wake-up plan.

Especially in these first few days, do your absolute best to stick with your new rules. If you have decided that your little one needs to stay in their room until the first wake-up after 3 AM, that's what happens. If they wake and call out from behind the gate or door strap or come to your room, tell them to get back in bed. Once they do, go in and sit in the chair. Make sure to point out that the wake-up light hasn't turned on / changed color yet (if you're using one). Stay until they're back asleep. Then make a point of mentioning the next day what a great job they did going back to sleep.

Be really boring.

In these first few days, you might be responding to waking a lot. Try to avoid saying much. You don't need to remind or explain. Your responses should be boring. Too much attention to the waking can reinforce it. It's going to be a challenge to stay neutral when it's the eighth time your live-wire is up that night. *"Omg, again? I literally just got you to sleep. Please just stay in bed!"* All that does is make you frustrated and furious, and it probably causes your livewire to be more awake. Instead, take a breath and then act like you've just been shot full of Novocain or that you are made of rubber. I used to think of it as being really floppy. If you can detach from your own exasperation, it's going to save you a lot of emotional wear and tear and help you avoid those terrible feelings of regret for losing it. Be floppy. Be boring.

Use the wake-up clock.

If you are using a wake-up clock (which we absolutely recommend), point to the clock when returning them to bed to remind them that it's not on yet, so it's still time for sleeping. A wake-up clock can also be handy if you have set a time for when it's okay to come into your room to the floor bed. You can have it turn on at whatever time you've agreed on.

What to do about early rising (before 6 AM)

Early rising is a common by-product of messing with familiar patterns and can be common during the sleep coaching process. Here's how to deal with it in the moment:

> **Set the wake-up clock for 6 AM.** A wake-up clock can be really helpful in reinforcing that it's still time to stay in bed when they're ready to start the day at 5 AM. Set it no earlier than 6 AM.

Wait until 6 AM to start the day. If they wake a lot earlier than 6 AM, treat it as a night waking and coach them back to sleep. If it's fairly close to 6 AM, see if they will hang out for a bit on their own until their wake-up clock's light turns on. If they instead make a ruckus, go in, remind them that it's not time to get up until the light turns on, and sit in your chair. Don't leave the room until 6 AM.

If they don't go back to sleep. Once their wake-up light turns on, you can say, "The light turned on! Time to get up!" If you're not using a clock, you can instead use what Kim calls a Dramatic Wake-Up: Leave the room briefly (count to ten or twenty) and then come back in and turn on the light with a bright, "Okay! Good morning! Time to get up!" This little bit of playacting sends the message that *you* have decided to start the day and it's not connected to them staying awake (though it totally is).

Make sure to write your plan for early rising into your Change the Pattern Worksheet. If the early rising starts happening every day and shows no signs of budging, refer to page 263 for how to assess and address it.

Days Four to Six: Position Two (At the Door)

Day Four is when you make your first move. In her book *The Sleep Lady's Good Night, Sleep Tight*, Kim recommends moving straight from beside the bed to at the door inside the room, skipping the middle-of-the room position that we use for younger kiddos, because it tends to reduce the power struggle (climbing into your lap, pulling you to come to the bed, etc.) you may run into at this distance. However, if you have a livewire who really, really needs a gradual approach and you want to use a middle step, that's fine. You will be at this middle ground for Days Four to Six and move to the door for Days Seven to Nine.

Overview of This Position
BEDTIME

- Review the Bedtime Chart during the day to give your child a heads-up about what's happening that night, including where you'll be sitting.
- Have a good pre-routine routine and a solid, consistent bedtime routine.
- Check items off the chart as you go.
- Move your chair *to the door* and use only your voice to calm.
- If they get really upset, use a hug to help calm them. Once they're calm, return to your chair.
- Stay until they're completely asleep.

WAKE-UPS

- If they're supposed to stay in their room, walk them back to their bed and let them get themselves back in and under the covers.
- If you're using a wake-up clock, point to it and remind them that it's still time to sleep.
- Return to your chair and stay until they're completely asleep.

THE NEXT DAY

- Remember to review the Bedtime Chart and any progress the next morning.
- Give lots of attention to what went well and ignore what didn't.

BEDTIME AND WAKE-UPS: WHAT TO DO AND HOW TO AVOID CURVEBALLS

On Day Four, you will move your chair to the door but remain inside the room. If you have gone a little slower, that's fine. The key is just to *move every two or three days*. Otherwise, you can get stuck in that position and the next move can feel a little like starting over.

Day Four can be bumpy.

It's important to know that on Day Four, protest can tick up again. The fourth day is typically when your child will make one last push to get things to go back to the way they were before. Continue to be supportive, but keep going. The resistance should mellow out on Day Five and beyond. Don't let Day Four throw you.

Rehearse, rehearse, rehearse.

Consider rehearsing this change during the day on Day Four. Have your child get in bed, pretending like it's bedtime, and show them where the chair is going to be. Let them know that you will still be there until they're asleep, but their job is to learn how to go to sleep without back rubs, holding your hand, etc.

Hold the line on bedtime shenanigans.

Continue to hold those limits on shenanigans: Use if/when statements, and use the baby gate or door strap as a boundary.

You can still hug to calm them.

Throughout this process, you can always hug to calm. Hopefully, the worst of the protest will have passed. If it hasn't and they get worked up, you can always hug them to calm them down and then go back to where you were in the chair.

Keep a close eye on "last" requests.

Be vigilant about any small requests for a last tuck-in or hug. These seemingly innocuous asks can trip progress up. You give in to one, and suddenly the requests become more frequent or start looking like they're now part of the go-to-sleep ritual. Make sure you write all the "lasts" into the chart. When they're done, they're done.

Common What Ifs at This Position

"What if my child just comes up to me and begs me to come back to being closer?"

Continuing to move away is key if you don't want to be trapped in your child's room forever. We *have to* nudge them to get better at it. There are always going to be growing pains with this process, but you have to keep holding the line. What you're asking of them is reasonable, and what you're doing now is unsustainable. Remember, we're not helping their fears or worries by making accommodations (like moving back to sit by the bed when we were already away or turning on lights so they won't be scared). The only way children move through fears and worries is to face them gradually and with support. If pleading continues, don't get into a big discussion. Simply use the if/when strategy again: *"If you choose to keep asking, I will go sit in the hallway on the other side of the gate. When you are back in bed / quiet, I'll sit in my chair by the door again."*

"What if my child seems to stay awake to keep checking that I'm there?"

This is tricky and also *very* common. I've worked with a lot of livewires who will keep themselves awake to make sure their parent hasn't left. Alertness, persistence, perceptiveness, and zero desire to sleep all converge into this challenging "checking" behavior. Persistent checking can be a response to the potential of you leaving, especially if you used to leave before they were asleep. The good news is that you're *not* going to leave until they are completely asleep. Chronic checking will hopefully mellow out as they see that you are staying consistent and keeping your word about staying.

Make sure you've discussed this when making the bedtime chart and consider putting it in the chart as a step for *you* to do: *"I [parent] will stay in my chair inside the door until you are asleep."*

You can also practice short separations during the day. For example, if you're going to read to them, you could say, *"I forgot to get my glasses,*

I'll be right back" or *"I need to visit the bathroom. I'll be back in just a couple of minutes."* Leave briefly and then return. Games like hide-and-seek can also help them practice being physically separate and out of sight for brief periods.

If you feel that the constant checking looks less like age-appropriate separation worry and more like anxiety or hypervigilance, and it's also starting to happen at other times during the day, get professional input and assessment.

Days Seven to Nine: Position Three (Outside the Door but in View)

Overview of This Position
BEDTIME

- Review the Bedtime Chart during the day to give them a heads-up about what's happening that night, including where you'll be sitting.
- Have a good pre-routine routine and a solid, consistent bedtime routine.
- Check items off the chart as you go.
- Move your chair *out into the hallway (or other side of the gate), but still in view.*
- From here, you are only using your voice to soothe.
- If they get really upset, use a hug to help them calm down (sparingly). Once they're calm, return to your chair.
- Stay until they're completely asleep.

WAKE-UPS

- If they're supposed to stay in their room, walk them back to bed and let them get themselves back in and under the covers.
- If you're using a wake-up clock, point to it and remind them that it's still time to sleep.
- Return to your chair and stay until they're asleep again.

THE NEXT DAY

- Remember to review the Bedtime Chart and any progress the next morning.
- Give lots of attention to what went well and ignore what didn't.

BEDTIME AND WAKE-UPS:
AVOIDING CURVEBALLS

Once you make a move to outside the door, kids in beds really feel the separation. Even though they may have been getting the hang of falling asleep without you right there, once you are outside the room, separation worries rise to the surface. If they didn't have a big bump up in struggle on Day Four, they might now, when they realize that you're not going to be inside the room anymore. This is okay and normal. Below are some strategies that can help you keep going. If you can't have the door all the way open because too much light gets in, make sure you still crack the door enough that they can see you.

Rehearse, rehearse, rehearse.

Do a quick run-through of this position during the day so that your child gets a feel for what it will be like. Technically, this isn't a lot different from sitting right by the door, but if you're using a gate, you will now be on the other side of it. That can be a bit of a game-changer for your livewire. So, give them a heads-up before bedtime and have them test it out.

Continue to offer reassurance before the light goes out.

Remind them that even though you're in the hall, you're still there and you will stay until they're asleep. Tell them that you believe in their ability to take this next step.

Stay confident and strong yourself.

Being outside the room is an important step. If you don't want to be stuck in the room waiting for them to go to sleep forever, you really have to master this move. I know that this is where parents commonly get caught because their livewire loses it when they're outside the doorway. Hopefully, with rehearsals, preparation, warnings, and reminders, your livewire won't be quite so blindsided. This is a crucial step for everyone. Push through the pushback that might come with this position.

I've heard lots of parents of persistent two- or three-year-olds say, "I've tried, but they won't *let me* leave the room." This is a surefire sign that the parents have very little fight left in them and feel like their small child is the one in charge. If you've said this yourself (I know I have), it means you need to double down on your commitment to following this process. *You* are driving the bus, and your livewire needs to get on board.

Days Ten to Twelve: Position Four (Outside the Door and Out of View)

Overview of This Position
BEDTIME

- Review the Bedtime Chart during the day to give them a heads-up about what's happening that night, including where you'll be sitting.
- Have a good pre-routine routine and a solid, consistent bedtime routine.
- Check items off the chart as you go.
- Move your chair *out into the hallway out of view*. This could be just around the corner of the door. They should be able to hear you but not see you.
- Use only your voice from the hallway to soothe.
- As always, if they get really upset, use a hug to help them calm down. Once they're calm, return to your chair.
- Stay until they're completely asleep.

WAKE-UPS

- If they're supposed to stay in their room, walk them back and let them get themselves back in and under the covers. If they are calling for you from the bed, just go to the doorway and reassure from there.
- If you're using a wake-up clock, point to it and remind them that it's still time to sleep.
- Return to your chair in the hall and stay until they're asleep again.

THE NEXT DAY

- Remember to review the Bedtime Chart and any progress the next morning.
- Give lots of attention to what went well and ignore what didn't.

BEDTIME AND WAKE-UPS: HOW TO AVOID CURVEBALLS

Having their parent out of view can really be especially tricky for anxious livewires. However, it's important with anxiety of any kind that we don't get stuck accommodating it completely. We have to help our livewires get gradually better at handling that feeling of separation.

Don't get stuck "in view."

I've seen some parents get stuck having to stay where the child can still see them. I remember one dad who had to sit in the hallway so that just his feet were still visible. The minute he withdrew them (even while staying in the same spot), his daughter freaked out. A parent Kim worked with came up with a solution for this: Once the child was successfully staying in bed at bedtime, the parent would stuff their shoes with newspaper and just stick them in the doorway so they could finally leave. Ideally, you would then practice with gradually removing the shoes, but I would still call this a very creative win.

Rehearse, rehearse, rehearse.

This is the first position where you won't be in view. Practice this in the daytime for sure. You can even use a little game, like a variation of the animal sounds game that we mentioned for fear of the dark (page 156). Have your livewire lie on their bed in their room, and go into the hallway where they can't see you. Take turns making an animal sound and having the other person say what it is. This shows your child that you can still hear and respond to them even though they can't see you. Start by doing this in the daytime, and as they get better at it, try it in the early evening and then at a time when it's dark. (You might want to start this practice ahead of reaching this position, so they've already had some practice by the time you are out of view.)

Continue to offer reassurance before the light goes out.

Remind them that, even though you're in the hall and they can't see you, you're still there and you will stay until they're asleep. Tell them that you believe in their ability to take this next step.

Work toward being even farther away for wake-ups.

If your livewire is getting the hang of things, you don't have to return to the chair and stay until they're asleep. If they wake up and call out from their bed, you can reassure them from their doorway initially, then stay nearby for a bit before returning to your bed. Or, if your bedroom is close enough for them to hear you from there, can you verbally reassure from your bed?

Day Thirteen and Beyond: Position Five (Periodic Check-Ins)

Overview of This Position

BEDTIME

- Review the Bedtime Chart during the day to give them a heads-up about what's happening that night, including where you'll be sitting.
- Have a good pre-routine routine and a solid, consistent bedtime routine.
- Check items off the chart as you go.
- After you say good night, *leave the room and just check in periodically*.
- Tell them you will come back to check on them and make sure you do that until they're completely asleep.

WAKE-UPS

- If they wake up and they're supposed to stay in their room, remind them to go back and get themselves in bed. If you have to, walk them silently back to their room.
- If you're using a wake-up clock, point to it and remind them that it's still time to sleep.
- Once they are back in bed, leave again and check in periodically until they're completely asleep.

THE NEXT DAY

- Remember to review the Bedtime Chart and any progress the next morning.
- Give lots of attention to what went well and ignore what didn't.

BEDTIME AND WAKE-UPS: HOW
TO AVOID CURVEBALLS

Starting with Day Thirteen, you will be periodically checking in with your child until they fall asleep. Just go to the door (unless they're really crying and you think something is up, of course; then you can go in) and shush a bit.

You can decide how frequently these check-ins happen. You could do them at set time intervals (for example, every five minutes) or as needed. For vigilant older livewires, you can also try "job checks," which means you say good night and tell them that you're going to go—to clean the kitchen, put on your pajamas, run to the bathroom—and that you'll check in after that. If you find that your alert little one is waiting for you to return rather than going to sleep, make 100 percent sure that your check-in is completely uninteresting. Maybe you just pop your head in silently, or do a quick shush, so that it's underwhelming for them and not worth waiting for.

Hopefully, by this time, you have hit your stride and sleep is a lot better than it was before. If you have any challenges (waking before 6 AM?) that crop up or still seem stubborn, or you are stuck, chapter twelve will help you figure out where you veered off the map.

WORKBOOK TO DO

Make sure you add your notes from this chapter to your Sleep Plan Worksheet. Then, use all the notes you've made so far to fill out the Sleep Plan Road Map, which will be your guide for navigating this new process.

Let's Talk About Improving Naps (Finally!)

So far, we haven't really said anything about naps except "make sure you get enough of them." This is because getting *any* child to nap at this age can be tough, and with livewires—*yikes*. The reason we harp on naps is because getting enough naptime (which may not happen when you do nap coaching) really helps your work on nighttime.

It *is* possible that once nighttime skills kick in, naps will also get easier. We've seen it happen. I've also seen situations where even though parents get their livewire to sleep great at night, no amount of nap coaching made a dent in daytime behaviors. Some parents, once they are happy with the nighttime sleep, decide to just let naps be what they are.

Livewires at these older ages are also more likely than their mellower counterparts to drop their naps completely. Children technically need naps until at least four years. Dropping them earlier is not ideal, but with livewires, the work it takes to get them to nap is prohibitive (especially if you have another child at home). Or, if they nap at all, it destroys a reasonable bedtime. Parents commonly tell me, "If we let her nap even twenty minutes during the day, she won't fall asleep until 10 PM that night." Again, not ideal, but incredibly common for livewires.

One thing that can help is having the nap take place somewhere other than their bed. I've seen creative parents create a nap fort or nap tent where their livewire can get cozy. Feel free to try whatever you think will work for them to be able to fall asleep. If your livewire conks out great in the car during the ride home from preschool (and it's not too late in the day to affect bedtime), awesome. Sleep is sleep.

STRATEGIES FOR GETTING A NAP

If your livewire is still napping (or you think they could with some encouragement) and you are ready to work on independent nap skills, here are the basic steps. These are almost identical to what you will have done for bedtime. You'll just be applying those same skills to naps.

1. **Have a brief nap routine or transition time.** Give your livewire some transition time ahead of when their nap should start by lowering the lights or closing the blinds, maybe reading a story. If your livewire naps well at daycare but not at home, find out what they do to prepare for the nap. Is there a song they play? A routine they follow? Try to mimic at home what happens there. We cannot just expect them to go right from "full steam ahead" to "It's naptime!"

2. **Follow the steps you followed at bedtime.** However, here's how this differs: You will need to put a limit on how long you try to get them to nap. Otherwise, that nap delay will do a number on their ability to fall asleep at bedtime. An hour is what we usually suggest, but if that's too big an ask, choose an amount of time that you know you can stick to (*"I'll try for forty minutes"*). If there are shenanigans, use the if/when strategy to re-enforce that this is resting time, not playing time.

3. **Use their wake-up clock or a Dramatic Wake-Up to end the rest time.** You can use the wake-up clock to help them know when the nap attempt or Quiet Time is over. When the light turns on, you can say it's time to get up. If you're not using a clock and they don't fall asleep in the window you have set, leave the room, count to ten or twenty, and then come in with a bright "Okay! We're getting up!" to communicate that *you* are ending the nap attempt, not their delay or pushback.

4. **Have a backup plan.** You will have to decide if it's necessary to get them *some* sleep if they do not nap that day. You have two choices: (1) make bedtime earlier that evening, or (2) have a short backup nap strategy (a ride in the car or stroller, etc.) so that they're not a cranky basket case for their regular bedtime. You may decide it's enough for them to just power down for a little, midday, by listening to a recorded story or watching a quiet video.

5. **If they don't get a good nap or break, move bedtime earlier.** If your livewire still doesn't get adequate downtime during the day, make bedtime a little earlier so you aren't facing a double dose of overtiredness.

If your livewire is younger than four years, we really want this one nap to be longer than forty-five minutes. Once they've gotten the hang of falling asleep on their own at the start of naptime, you can use the same strategy if they wake up after just one sleep cycle (thirty or forty minutes). Set a time limit (e.g., thirty minutes) and try to coach them back to sleep. Even if they only go back to sleep for ten minutes, that's a win. The goal here is to get them to learn how to connect sleep cycles so that they're not waking up completely every time they move into light sleep.

Nap coaching can be a lot of work for the parents of *any* child. With livewires, oh boy. It can take a few weeks of dedication. As long as you're making progress, keep going, but also follow your gut. If your livewire is sleeping well at night, you may be able to lighten up on your nap work. If you've really tried with naps and you hit a dead end, this may have to be another "call it good" moment.

QUIET TIME AS AN ALTERNATIVE TO A NAP

For many children four years or so and up, it may not be critical for them to actually sleep during the day. Quiet Time can be an acceptable alternative. It's a brief period of quiet, nonstimulating activity that gives their brain a little time to decompress. For busy, headstrong three-year-old livewires, Quiet Time may be the best you can do.

Getting a livewire to spend time being *quiet . . . by themselves . . .* in their room sounds like a massive task all by itself. And it can be. But Quiet Time is a short sensory break, and it doesn't have to be long.

Here are some possible Quiet Time strategies:

- Create a Quiet Time fort or tent where they go only during this time. It can have pillows and stuffed animals.
- If you haven't already, as part of your transition, close the blinds or curtains and dim the lights. If possible, turn on special fairy lights or other colored lights that are only used for Quiet Time.
- Have your child listen to a recorded sleep visualization story (page 149) in their Quiet Time fort. Who knows? It might even help

them fall asleep! In the meantime, listening will engage their brain without the stimulation of visuals. You could also find other recorded stories (not specifically for sleep).

- Have quiet toys or activity books that only come out for Quiet Time.
- If necessary, a quiet video on the couch with lowered lights and blinds could even work.
- Use a wake-up clock to let them know when Quiet Time is done.

Really, *any* rest is better than no rest, and any reduced stimulation can help them reset a little.

CHAPTER 12

Sleep Triage 101: Uh-Oh . . . What If . . . ? What the . . . ?

How to Know If It's Working and What to Do When It's Not

Being able to assess whether old patterns are budging is going to be a lifeline in this process. Past sleep training disasters may have left you so, so skeptical that anything will work. We need to make sure you can spot those glimmers of traction and keep going. Livewires rarely will give you giant neon signs of victory, but if you know where to look, you will find positive signs along this bumpy road.

THE IMPORTANCE OF KEEPING A SLEEP LOG

Keeping a sleep log is going to be critical in helping you assess whether you're making headway. This log is going to be essential for you to be able to detect not only progress but also patterns and relationships in your livewire's sleep behaviors.

For example, if a night was unexpectedly bad, check their wake windows and nap amounts for the day. Were they overtired? If you find that, yes, they were under on naptime and were awake too long at some point, you have just learned an important piece of data: Your livewire is sensitive to not getting adequate sleep during the day.

The log will also show you changes in how many wake-ups there were, how long it takes them to fall asleep, etc. Trust me on this: You will want to be able to see change. When you are exhausted and hopeless, seeing even a little improvement is going to give you a boost.

WHAT PROGRESS LOOKS LIKE

To know if you're at all on the right track in Days One to Three, you're going to want to see *something* move:

- How long it took to fall asleep
- How difficult it was to get them to sleep
- How hard they protested (Were there breaks in the intensity or duration of crying?)
- How many wake-ups there were
- Any longer stretches between wake-ups
- Any wake-ups that were a little shorter
- Any sign that your child woke but put themselves back to sleep

Look carefully at your log and compare the first two nights. *Any* improvement in *any* of the behaviors is a win. If on the third night you see other changes (even if they're different ones), that's a clear indication that you are on the right path and that you are having an impact.

Here's another important caveat:

Progress does not happen in a straight line with livewires.

For dandelion sleepers, the process mostly looks like this:

Hard → better → better → better → better → solved!

For livewires, it's more like:

Awful → little better → little better →
Oops, what? That was working! What happened? →
Okay, that's better → What the . . . ? →
OMG, that was awful →
Woo-hoo! They slept through! →
They slept through *again*! →
Wait, why are they up at 1 AM? →
Solved (mostly)!

You unfortunately can't expect progress to be consistent or linear for livewires. When we start monkeying with their patterns, it can cause ripple effects that we didn't anticipate. Something that was good starts getting worse, or something that *was* working stops working. Nighttime gets better, then naps start to tank. Don't think of this as a sign you're doing something wrong or that you should stop. That's where you may have gotten stuck before. *Just keep going. Typically* (and I use that word loosely because live-wires rarely follow a typical pattern), bedtime gets easier first and then night wake-ups become shorter and/or fewer, then any early rising improves. Naps sometimes also improve at the same time. The morning ones improve first and then afternoon naps.

Even if you really feel like it's all over the place—and it might be—that's okay. Remember, as long as *you* are doing what you need to be doing, change and how fast it's happening are up to them. The only thing you can control is your own behavior and what you are or aren't doing to facilitate sleep. We can't *make* them go to sleep or stay asleep. All we can do is keep an eye on what *we* are doing in response. These little guys can be stubborn. I've had clients where we see improvement, but one piece (like a certain waking) just won't budge—then just when we think it's not going to happen, it falls into place.

The first few days are so important. If you see even a *little* change from Day One to Day Two, and then *any* change from Day Two to Day Three, you are in good shape. Most of the changes happen in the first four to seven days. If you can really commit to being on your game in this first stage of work, the rest of the process will be much easier.

HOW TO KNOW WHETHER YOU TOOK A WRONG TURN AND HOW TO GET BACK ON TRACK

Let's say you got started, and things seemed to be going well; you were seeing progress. Then . . . that progress stopped. Most of the popular sleep books lack a critically important piece of information that parents of live-wires need: *what to do if it doesn't go as planned.* Sleep experts tend to over-simplify how their method will work and overpromise on the results—at least as far as livewires are concerned. The books typically say something like, "Just do A, B, and C, and in about a week, your child will be sleeping through!" But what if it's not just "a few nights" and nothing—not A, not B, and *definitely* not C—worked? What then? Rarely do you get guidance about what to do beyond "Just do A, B, and C harder."

We're going to give you some of the tools we use as coaches of livewires of all ages to assess problems that crop up or improvement that slows down or stalls. Most importantly, we're going to give you ideas for what to do if sleep isn't budging at all. Remember, we don't want you banging your head against the wall when there's something standing in the way. We'll help you become a sleep triage ninja.

FIRST, REVISIT THE BIG FOUR

Any time sleep behavior or progress gets wobbly or stalls, first revisit the Big Four sleep tankers. Sometimes, with livewires, it doesn't take much to trip everything up, and it's good to make sure that at least all *your* ducks are in a row.

Start by looking at your sleep log and your livewire's sleep targets for nap amount, wake windows, and nighttime sleep. Then, ask yourself the following:

Sleep Tanker #1 (Overtiredness): Did you hit their sleep targets / avoid their second wind yesterday?

Sleep Tanker #2 (Problematic lead-up to lights out): How was the bedtime routine? Was the lead-up to lights out the same as it had been up until the previous night?

Sleep Tanker #3 (You are part of the go-to-sleep pattern): Have you been good about consistently reducing how much you are participating in their go-to-sleep pattern? Were they drowsier than you thought when you put them in bed?

Sleep Tanker #4 (Inconsistency): Were you consistent with what you were supposed to be doing at this point in the process? (Did you do a little more touching / holding / singing than you usually do? After a lot of work, did you end up doing what you used to, to get them to sleep? Did you go back to the side of the crib / bed too much or too often once you were "away"?)

If you answered no to any of these, don't stress. This is a big lift, and some missteps do not mean you have "failed" or have to start over. Say something nice to yourself and get back up on the horse. You may have to back up a step for a few days before moving forward again, but chalk it up to learning.

Now, let's dive deeper together into figuring out how things veered off track.

Is the culprit "overtired / wired"?

How were naps and awake windows? If bedtime or nighttime are tanking or not improving, the *first* area to look at is naps (timing and quantity) and bedtime (timing). Did your livewire hit their nap targets? Did they stay within their max awake window? Was bedtime well-timed based on their naps and the time they got up for the day? Was the last nap *too* close to bedtime? If your livewire is no longer napping, was bedtime later than you wanted?

If naps or bedtime were off, see what you can do to hit those targets more squarely the next day and assess whether that affects nighttime sleep. Some parents have to be perfectly on target or else bedtime / nighttime is a total circus. Others may have a tiny bit of wiggle room. This will be helpful information when deciding how strict you need to be with naps and bedtime.

If everything was on track with regard to timing, look at the next sleep tanker: problems with the lead-up to lights out.

Is the culprit problems with the pre-routine or bedtime routine? Were they drowsier than you thought? Being *too* drowsy at bedtime is a big monkey wrench and may not be as obvious as it sounds. Remember, "drowsy" in little ones doesn't mean "half-asleep." Livewires can *look* totally awake even when their brain is already halfway to sleep. If they fall asleep in less than ten or fifteen minutes in the early part of this working-on-sleep process, they were already halfway to Sleepytown by the time they hit the mattress. Parents often think that it's a good thing when their little one falls asleep superfast. But it's actually a very sneaky fly in the old ointment.

Remember, in this early phase of working on sleep skills, we *want* your livewire to grapple a little with the go-to-sleep process. A child that is 80 percent of the way to sleep when they get in bed is likely to need help getting back to that 80 percent mark when they wake at night. We actually want them going into the crib or bed only 10 to 20 percent drowsy, so they are going nearly the *whole* way on their own. Then, when they wake at night, they will have a road map for how to get *all the way* back to sleep on their own. We want to get them in bed *awake,* even if that means getting them to sleep will be harder at first than it is right now.

Ask yourself whether you have slid into allowing your child to be drowsier than they should be or you did just a little more touching because it makes things *so much easier*. The lure of "easier" is strong. I get it. You may be a little wiped out from the first week of coaching and have inadvertently let your child get a *little* droopy before they go into the crib. Or you knew if you just rocked for *thirty seconds*, it would cut the falling asleep time in half. Or you rubbed their back "just a little" and then they fall asleep "so fast." Watch out because this will bite you in the middle of the night. We need your child to be awake at bedtime so that when they wake up at 2 AM, they know how to get *all* the way back without that extra help from you.

Were they too awake? Alternatively, were they *too* awake at bedtime? Did they have enough time to decompress during the bedtime routine? Did they still have a chunk of physical or mental energy they had to offload? Was their last nap a little late and they weren't able to build enough sleep pressure for bedtime? You don't want them trying to decompress once the lights are out or starting the negotiation show simply because they're not ready for sleep.

Is the culprit sneaky issues with their go-to-sleep pattern?
Are *you* still part of that pattern? There can be teeny tiny actions—as parents, we may not even notice them—that can throw a monkey wrench into the go-to-sleep process. If you are at the point where you have moved away from the crib or bed (Day Four on), take a close look at exactly what you are doing as your livewire is falling asleep at bedtime. Have there been any last bits of touching (when you're "away" from the crib or bedside)? Remember, little actions can accidentally get knitted into the new pattern. To you, a final little kiss or going crib- or bedside for a quick back pat may be almost nothing, but your child has now incorporated it into their go-to-sleep pattern (which is the same as their middle-of-the-night back-to-sleep pattern). If you don't want to have to give "one more kiss" at 2 AM, don't do it at bedtime.

Has there been *any* inconsistency? Remember, with livewires, you have to be almost rigid in your consistency—especially early in the process. We're saying this again and again because for tired, stressed-out livewire parents whose tanks are almost on empty, consistency is *hard*. We get it. But it's inconsistency that makes the process *so much* harder and absolutely kneecaps your efforts. When you look *very* carefully at your actions, have there been *any* differences in your actions night to night? Or parent to parent? Remember, if you have been wobbly in the past, you may need to be even *more* consistent over a *longer* period to show your perceptive livewire that you are committed and will hold the line.

Have you gotten stuck in one position? Sometimes parents accidentally get stuck in one spot for longer than three days. While it can be okay to tack on one more day to a position to really solidify a skill, you don't want to stay for much longer than that. The point of moving every few nights is to keep nudging the bar. If you stay in one place too long, that becomes the new normal, and then, once you *do* move, it can feel like starting over. If you've been next to the crib or bed for more than three or four days at bedtime, it's time to move. There might be a bump up in protest when you do this, but that should be temporary. Even when you are taking baby steps, it's critical that you *keep moving* toward doing less every few days.

TROUBLESHOOTING THE TRICKY SPOTS AND GETTING UNSTUCK

If you've assessed the Big Four and nothing really jumps out at you as problematic, there can be other gremlins getting in the way. With livewires, the road to better sleep is full of unexpected twists and turns, and new patterns rarely fall neatly (and linearly) into place.

Below are some common bumps in the sleep coaching road that often cause parents to abandon their efforts. We're not going to let that happen. You have done some hard, important work so far. Don't give up.

Some things have improved, others not so much.

First of all . . . yay! *Any* improvement is a sign that you are doing a good job, your part of the sleep equation is on point, and your livewire is responding. Parents often expect that everything will improve together in a nice gradual progression. But you're dealing with a livewire here. Some things will improve, and some will tank. Then those things will improve, and new pieces will fall apart. As long as *something* (anything) is moving, know that you are on the right track.

Bedtime still takes a long time.

No matter what you do, some livewires just take a million years to fall asleep. If you have set the stage appropriately for sleep and your livewire is talking or singing to themselves after lights out, that's technically okay—as long as you don't have to be there for it. We can't *make* children fall asleep. All we can do is lay a solid foundation and get out of the way. If you don't have to play a role in their go-to-sleep show, you can call that good.

However, if all of *your* bedtime tasks have been handled (enough naptime, good bedtime timing, good routine, no *you* in the go-to-sleep pattern) and falling asleep is still taking them an hour or more, with a lot of struggle to get comfortable or settle, revisit the physiological causes of sleep disruption in chapter four. A long time to fall asleep can be a sign of restless legs syndrome, obstructive sleep apnea, anxiety, food allergies, or other diagnosable causes.

Bedtime is good, but they're awake for two hours at night.

A split night (where a child is up for an hour or more in the middle of the night) can stem from either too little daytime sleep or, believe it or not, too much.

Too little naptime means they're on overdrive at bedtime, and the chemicals that were helping them stay awake can do a number on nighttime sleep. (You know what you're like when you've had too much caffeine. You can be tired and still completely unable to sleep.) Look at your livewire's nap targets and compare them to what they're getting now. If they're low on naptime, or they're spending long periods awake during the day, spend a few days redoubling efforts to fill up that nap tank and see if it causes that split night to budge.

On the other hand, if they are napping *too much* (I know, *What's this "too much naptime" thing you're talking about?*), it could be eating into their nighttime sleep budget. Children can only sleep so much in twenty-four hours, and champion nappers could be using up some of what they should be getting at night. In these rare cases, try capping their naps to more closely hit the target.

If naps are on target (not too long, not too short) and this kind of wake-up is *still* happening, it could be an indicator of either obstructed breathing or low ferritin. Take another look at chapter four to see if any of the other symptoms are present.

They're still crying at bedtime.

The first one of the Big Four we look at in this situation is overtiredness. An overtired / wired child will be crankier at bedtime. If naps and bedtime are on track and there are no other signs of physical discomfort like teething or oncoming illness, it's possible that your livewire just needs to blow off some steam before they go to sleep.

We don't want them crying hard for a long time, of course, but parents usually have a gut instinct about whether the crying at bedtime is a signal of pain or just their livewire's way of downshifting to sleep. If you have done *everything* you can to set them up for sleep success *and* the crying has gotten shorter over time *and* they aren't hysterical, it may be just something they do. Kim worked with a toddler who, no matter what the parents did, would stand up at bedtime, throw all her things out of the crib, scream for a couple of minutes—and then plop down and go to sleep. The mom ultimately felt that her child just needed to have the last word.

They're suddenly waking up at 5 AM every day.

Early rising (any waking for the day earlier than 6 AM) is sometimes merely an artifact of learning a new sleep skill. When little ones are learning about sleep, all kinds of patterns can go a little haywire. It's possible that this will resolve as your livewire gets the hang of sleeping more solidly. However, if they've been falling asleep independently, sleeping well at night, but this early rising is still happening, here's how to ferret out the cause.

There are several potential causes of early rising:

1. Too little naptime
2. Too late a bedtime
3. Too big a gap between naps or between the last nap and bedtime
4. Going into the crib or bed too drowsy
5. Hunger (if your child is an infant and you've been trying to completely night wean, they may still really need one feed overnight)
6. Snoring or mouth breathing (sleep apnea is a sneaky cause of early rising)

Take a look at your sleep logs to see if any of these could be a culprit.

Once you figure out the problem, however, know that early rising can be stubborn. Even when all the pieces are in place, resolving it can take some time and Olympic-caliber consistency on your part. Just keep going.

Strategies for handling early wake-ups

Early rising can be hard on parents, and how much you can do about it really depends on your child's age. You want to make sure that you are addressing the underlying causes during the day, of course, but when you're *in* that early-morning moment, you have a few choices for addressing it, depending on what you think you can get away with.

For infants under a year, try a quick feed. If they've slept straight through from 7 PM to 5 AM, they may be hungry, as discussed earlier.

A quick feed may get you a little more sleep before you have to get up. You can phase this out when they're a little older.

For toddlers and up, use a wake-up clock to let them know when it's time to get up. Older children (three and up) may be able to entertain themselves if they wake before a certain time.

Coach them back down. If it's not time for them to wake up and there's no feed scheduled or needed, do whatever you have been doing at bedtime and other wake-ups to coach them back to sleep. For toddlers, point to the wake-up clock (if you're using one) and say, "The clock hasn't changed color / turned on. It's still nighttime." (Be sure to include this expectation on your sleep chart: "I stay in my bed quietly until the light changes color / turns on.")

Use a Dramatic Wake-Up. If you are still trying to coach them back to sleep when it's time to start the day, don't just get them out of the crib or bed. Remember, if you've been coaching and coaching and then just give up and take them out of the room, your sharp livewire will connect their prolonged protest with getting taken out of the crib or bed and starting the day. You'll have inadvertently given them an incentive to just wait you out. Instead, use a Dramatic Wake-Up: Leave the room, count to ten, and come back in with a big, bright, "Okay! Time to get up!"

Brew the coffee. For some livewires, thinking you can get them to go back to sleep at that hour is wishful thinking. When these livewires are up, they are *up*, and no amount of coaching (or pleading) will get them back to sleep. They are ready and raring to go. Sometimes your only choice is to start the day. If this happens, see page 123 for ways to make up for that lost sleep during the day.

They wake up screaming in the middle of the night.

This can be so scary. Waking up to a child at a full scream always gets the adrenaline going. There are a few reasons why children wake out of a sound sleep like this.

Confusional arousals. Confusional arousals originate in the brain as it comes out of very deep sleep.[64] Part of the brain wakes up while the other part is still asleep. Children experiencing a confusional arousal may cry out, moan, or thrash around. *They are not actually awake.* You don't have to try to rouse them out of it or do a lot to calm them down. Intervening too much may prolong the episode.

Night terrors. Night terrors are a kind of confusional arousal that occurs in the first two or three hours after falling asleep and generally happens in children older than eighteen months.[65] Night terrors are not nightmares. In a night terror, your child isn't awake (even though their eyes might be open). You can usually tell that they're not aware of you or their surroundings, and when asked about it the next day, children typically don't even recall the event. This means that you don't have to wake them up or even try to intervene. They really are not awake. Night terrors can be a result of overtiredness. Your work on sleep timing and targets should address them, but if the terrors become more frequent or happen at the same time every night, it's something to talk to a pediatrician about.

Nightmares. These mostly happen in children over three or four years and they occur later in the night than terrors.[66] Unlike night terrors, the child is clearly awakened by them and will remember the content of their dream and tell you about it if you ask. The trick with nightmares is to give comfort and support without overdoing it. Make sure you reassure them that it was a dream (though for big-brain livewires, just knowing it wasn't real may not be enough to comfort them). Remember, livewires are not great at distracting themselves. It's possible they will keep mentally replaying whatever scary image / person / event was in their dream. You can try helping them create an alternate story or image that they can focus on. If a nightmare keeps reoccurring or is related to a real-life scary event or trauma, get some professional input on the best way to address it.

Confusional arousals, night terrors, and nightmares can stem from diagnosable sleep disorders. They can also be quite normal by-products of development. If these events continue to occur even after your child is sleeping better, talk to your pediatrician or your local pediatric sleep clinic.

UNAVOIDABLE ROAD HAZARDS

It's a sad fact that sleep doesn't *stay* done. Life happens. Development happens. And sleep can get bumpy again. You will likely have to do some sleep coaching booster sessions from time to time (no one tells you that, do they?). The good news is that once you know how to get sleep on track, you also know how to get it *back* on track. Plus, when you use an approach that doesn't break your heart, it's not hard to use it again when sleep goes sideways. Here are a couple of mostly unavoidable ways that sleep can get thrown off.

Sickness, regressions, teething, and travel

When your child is sick, *of course* you need to do a little more to help them at night. When you travel, you may not be able to maintain the same sleeping arrangements you have at home. The key is to make modifications without going *all* the way back to square one.

If you have to make significant adjustments to your routine (your child was really sick and you needed to feed / hold to sleep, you needed to co-sleep on vacation, etc.), you may need to do a booster session of sleep coaching after things return to normal to remind your little one about the go-to-sleep pattern they mastered before. This time, you can skip through the positions a little faster—moving positions every night, for example, instead of every three.

TRAVEL TIPS

It's difficult, if not impossible, to keep routines fully intact during a vacation. However, here are a few helpful ideas.

- Stick to awake windows, and do your best to get your child the naptime that they need.
- Keep an eye on how much stimulation and novelty they take in each day and be sure to schedule naps and breaks so that bedtime isn't more of a rodeo than it has to be.
- Bring familiar sleep items from home: lovies, sheets, etc.

Potty training

Sometimes your livewire will need to use the bathroom during the bedtime routine, especially as they're learning how. However, "I have to go potty" is also a great strategy for delaying bedtime or getting your attention in the middle of the night. Make sure you fold a "last bathroom trip" into the bedtime routine (and Bedtime Chart), potentially having it as the last step before lights out. Or consider a diaper or Pull-Up at night while they're learning.

You may feel that it's confusing for them to still use a diaper at night when they aren't during the day. I get that. But most children potty train during the day first. The ability to stay dry all night is not really a skill you learn; it's hormonal and physiological. In her potty-training coach program, Kim doesn't recommend taking the nighttime diaper or Pull-Up away until a child wakes dry for *ten days* in a row. It's okay to go back to Pull-Ups or diapers overnight if overnight training is getting in the way of sleep progress. You can explain that their body is not ready to be dry all night and that's okay.

If you (or they) don't want to use a Pull-Up or diaper for nighttime and your livewire needs the potty overnight, you can escort them to the bathroom, but be as boring as possible. Stand outside the bathroom, looking away, or wait for them in their room. If your child is old enough to get to the bathroom themselves but it's too dark, consider a rope light or other lights that they could follow to the bathroom, and make sure there's a dim night-light in there for them. You could also put a little potty chair in their room. If you're finding that there are more requests for bathroom visits than you think are necessary, put a limit on how often they are allowed to go. For example, they can go once before midnight and once after 4 AM, and for other wake-ups, you will just coach them back to sleep.

ROAD CLOSED: WHAT IF YOU MADE NO PROGRESS AT ALL IN THE FIRST THREE DAYS?

First, *good for you* for really going for it. But if you've given it a solid shot for at least two or three days, and in that time, there was a tsunami of crying each day with no tangible sign of change, we have to hit pause. While I've said that it's important to push through the pushback (and it is), we don't want children crying for hours with no change.

> *If there's been no change over two or three nights and there was a ridiculous amount of struggle each night, stop and reassess.*

The first step is to double-check the Big Four (overtiredness, not enough lead-up to bedtime, too drowsy at bedtime, and inconsistency). If those are on track, let's look at what else can cause this kind of roadblock.

There's an underlying physiological condition that you haven't identified yet.

When behavioral efforts appear to be a no go, physical pain or discomfort (oncoming illness, undiagnosed food intolerance, reflux, low ferritin levels, sleep apnea, etc.) is a common culprit. Check in with your gut feelings and revisit the list of physiological sleep disruptors and their symptoms in chapter four. Because you gave a behavioral approach such a solid try, you can now go to your pediatrician with the knowledge that the source of the problem isn't purely behavioral.

> ## NO WORK IS WASTED
>
> Even if you have to stop and get something checked out, keep whatever successful work you were able to do (fixing the sleep schedule, filling the nap tank, changing the go-to-sleep pattern, etc.). You can keep going with those while you try to figure out the rest.

There were previous false starts.

If you've tried several approaches unsuccessfully before—and you tried them in succession—your livewire just may not know which end is up. A sequence of attempts where you gave up and reverted to feeding, bouncing, or co-sleeping can stoke *much* higher levels of distress the next time you try anything because change and lack of predictability can throw livewires more than mellower children.

In these cases, you may need to start more slowly and have extreme levels of consistency and patience because you are, in a way, needing to undo all the previous methods and attempts. If you tried cry it out and stopped, then tried pick up, put down, then just packed it in and laid with them, you will need to be consistent with this new plan for a much longer period before your livewire will trust that this process is going to stick.

You took on too much too fast.

If you attempted to go from bouncing your livewire to sleep or lying in bed with them right to step 1 of the Shuffle, it may have been too big of a lift for your child. Consider whether there are smaller steps you can take first (for example, bounce to sleep again, but gradually bounce less over a few days, then try again for the crib after that, or sit up in your three-year-old's bed, then sit on the floor, etc.). If you were sure that your two-year-old was ready for a bed and it was a disaster, it's not a defeat to go back to a crib. It's not that sleep coaching didn't work. It's possible your livewire just was not ready for what you asked them to do.

It's also possible that you took on too much of the night. Maybe it was just more than you bargained for based on your current stamina level. Goodness knows, that's just a reality. You could pare down how much of the night you take on. If you were planning on coaching at bedtime *and* all night, maybe instead *just* work on bedtime and do what works the rest of the night. You could swap nursing or feeding with rocking back to sleep for now. You may find that focusing on only one battle is more doable. And remember, the secret sauce of this work is consistency. It's better to pick one piece you *know* you can solidly tackle than take on too much and be wobbly with it.

HOW TO KNOW WHEN IT'S SOMETHING "MORE"

Sometimes there is more going on than "just sleep problems." Nighttime fears are starting to really take over. Meltdowns are becoming frequent and feel unmanageable. Parts of the routine need to be redone a million times before they're "right." How do you know when it's time to consult a professional about your concerns? The following is a framework that was originally created to assess the need to intervene with anxiety,[67] but that I think is an effective way to assess a variety of challenges:

Disproportion: Is the behavior excessive and out of proportion to the situation or trigger?

Disruption: Does the behavior significantly interfere with daily life (mealtimes, daycare, sleep, etc.)? Does it happen in *more than one context* (for example, not just at home or not just at bedtime)?

> **Distress:** Does the behavior negatively affect your child? Does it negatively impact you as a parent (frustration, desperation, exhaustion, etc.)?
>
> **Duration:** Has it been going on for a while?
>
> **Durability:** Does the behavior persist even after you've done everything you think you can do as a parent?
>
> If your gut is telling you that your child's behavior is about something more than just their go-to-sleep patterns, do not hesitate to contact a clinical or medical provider (and don't take "you just have to sleep train" for an answer).

BECOMING A SLEEP PROBLEM TRIAGE NINJA

The key to being able to manage your livewire's sleep long-term is knowing which parts of the process belong to *you* and which ones belong to *your livewire*. You are in control of only a short list of factors: managing the timing and amount of sleep, establishing bedtime routines, and being consistent with what you are doing as they fall asleep and when they wake up at night. Understanding that list means that when sleep has gotten off track, you have a road map for how to get it back on course.

It also means that, as long as you are doing all of these things consistently, you can rule *yourself* out as the cause of any sleep issues. When I talk to parents who are on point with their part of their child's sleep and there are *still* big issues, it often means there's an underlying cause that needs investigation.

Sleep isn't an exact science. There may be times when you can't figure out what's happening, but with the tools we've discussed here, you are going to be able to identify and fix *most* of them. Livewires really march to their own drummer. As parents, the best we can do is to figure out what parade they're in and then get out in front of it.

OUR TRIP CHECKLIST

☑ You know you are on a different path.

☑ You understand your livewire's temperament strengths and challenges.

☑ You understand the link between temperament and sleep issues.

☑ Your child is ready:

    ☑ Over six months

    ☑ No upcoming disruptions

    ☑ No physiological issues that affect sleep

☑ You are ready (or as ready as you can be).

☑ You understand the Big Four sources of sleep issues.

☑ Big Strategy #1: You know how to avoid that second wind.

☑ Big Strategy #2: You have a solid, consistent bedtime routine.

☑ Big Strategy #3 and #4: You know how to change the go-to-sleep and back-to-sleep patterns and are prepared to be more consistent than you've ever been before.

☑ You know how to track progress.

☑ You know how to diagnose and fix any problems that arise.

☐ BETTER SLEEP!

The Parenting Road Is Long—Pack Snacks

CHAPTER 13

Blisters, Bumps, and Scrapes: This Is the Ironman of Parenting

Once you and your livewire start sleeping better, you may feel like you've summited a very big mountain . . . and you have. *Please* celebrate any and all victories, big or small. You absolutely 100 percent deserve it. Think of what you have already done and faced. Think of all the effort you have already put into not only improving your child's sleep but also understanding your child and yourself. You haven't just slain the dragons of overwhelming fatigue. You've put out a thousand meltdown fires. You have answered more questions than any human should have to. You are shepherding your miraculous livewire through these early years in a way that leaves their talents and true nature intact. You, my dear parent, are a hero.

You probably already know that your work isn't done once your livewire is sleeping. As moms who are much farther down this road, Kim and I can attest that temperament doesn't go away. Parenting a livewire can be a long, long road. At times, it's a little like parenting Whack-A-Mole—you resolve one issue, but there's another one (or four) coming in hot just around the bend. Or you finally sort of get the hang of one stage just as your little one is off to the next, and you're back to feeling like a rookie at this parenting game.

This is a path of extreme-sport-level growth. Raising a livewire is the Ironman Triathlon of parenting. And as much as you may sometimes secretly hope there is one, there's no off-ramp on this path, no frontage road that's just a tad less stressful.

Which is exactly why all of Section Five is devoted to *you* as a parent of a livewire. Because, unlike with the Ironman competition, you don't always get an advance warning that you're even *in* the race. You may not feel prepared, and you definitely haven't trained for an event of this size. And yet, there you are with a number on your arm.

Having a livewire impacts you on every level, and pretending that it's no different from any other parenting experience would be wrong. We know from research, from talking to parents of livewires, and from personal experiences that this road hits you on levels you didn't expect. We're going to talk about that so you know how much of this is normal for parents of a livewire. But the fact that you're *in* this race also means you are going to have to know how to keep yourself healthy and hydrated. This is about the long game. Pace yourself.

REMEMBER: YOU ARE NOT JUST A PARENTING PEZ DISPENSER

Parenting advice almost always focuses *exclusively* on you as a neutral dispenser of parenting strategies—as if you don't really exist as a living, breathing, exhausted vehicle for said strategies. And it always sounds so cut and dried when you read it—like a simple script that gets easy results: *"Honey, if you choose to just keep getting out of bed, I will have to leave the room."* Seems plausible, doesn't it? You can almost picture a little one saying "Okay, Mama," and peacefully getting back under the covers.

However, if this is the eightieth time you've said this today and you've had no sleep for the past, oh, three years, it's not going to come out like this. It may sound more like, *"Please, for the love of all that is holy, stay . . . in . . .*

bed . . . and . . . go . . . to . . . sleep! Mommy has had a really hard day, and she's very tired . . ." (It devolves from there.)

No one talks about how these scripts appear to have been written in a parenting vacuum where *you* don't exist as an entity with a history and values and experiences and mind-numbing fatigue and . . . um, your *own* temperament. You are not a parenting Pez dispenser. Parents are not neutral players in this parenting game. Everything we do and everything we say is filtered through our current and past experiences.

No one makes it through parenting little livewires without battle scars. We know, of course, that our livewires are stunningly amazing little humans and that every bit of effort is worth it. But it's just as important to acknowledge how hard this is, how much you are striving—and that you might feel traumatized from all the crying and sleepless nights you've experienced. I used to panic when my baby daughter would start to cry, *months* after colic had subsided, and even now, thirty years on, I still feel a bit of it rise up again when I hear a baby crying in the grocery store. I'm not bringing this up to be a downer. Instead, it's to let you know that we *all* have hit a variety of walls and fallen into emotional black holes—many, many times.

CHALLENGES UNIQUE TO PARENTS OF LIVEWIRES

All parents work super hard. Parenting any child can be exhausting and overwhelming. However, parenting a livewire comes with a few additional bombshells that require an even larger outlay of parenting energy and skill.

So much interaction

Livewires want us and need us . . . all . . . the . . . time. Even when they're tiny, they just don't seem into those great play mats or mobiles or really anything that's not a human face. When they're older, their brains and bodies can go a mile a minute with activity and questions and ideas and stories and comments about life. It's incredible, but it's a lot.

Many parents of livewires report that their little one just won't play on their own . . . ever. They need *you*; they want *you*. And when this level of interaction is required all day and doesn't stop at bedtime (or three in the morning), it can drain your energy tank right quick.

Feeling "touched out"

In addition to verbal interaction, livewires can require a lot of physical contact . . . like, *a lot*. Lots of nursing, lots of holding, lots of full-body contact—all day, at bedtime, and maybe all night. We know livewires need more help with regulating emotions, and going to sleep is hard . . . but oh boy. No wonder you just need them to go the heck to sleep at bedtime. You just want to have your own body back for two seconds.

This level of on-demand physical and emotional contact can lead to what author Susan Maushart calls *nurture shock*[68]—the feeling that your body is not your own, and instead, you're just a big cloud of "What do you need?" No one tells you about this before you become a parent. I know that it took me by surprise. It can be hard, if not impossible, to figure out how to get some my-own-body time. Don't worry. In chapter fourteen, we're going to help you prioritize and make a plan for shoring up your personal reserves.

Auditory bombardment

Parents can also become wiped out by the sheer volume and quantity of *sound* that comes with livewire parenting. Intense and persistent crying, meltdowns, even loud playing, singing, and talking can drain energy reserves and feel triggering to some parents.

Listening to a crying baby is a physiological event. Parents are wired to experience a baby's crying as negative and urgent (meaning, you don't want to listen to it for very long). When a baby cries, the parental nervous system goes on high alert. Evolutionarily, this is a good thing: Babies and young children quickly get the care they need. But when parents' internal alarms are going off *all the time* because there is so much freak-out, parents can feel desperate to just *make the crying or yelling stop*. We are not wired to be constantly triggered. This is the point where parents will do *anything* to avoid igniting a meltdown—not because they're "weak" or "permissive" but because their internal alarm system is burned to a crisp. If this is you, first, cut yourself some slack. Then read chapter fourteen for ways to prioritize and shore up your energy reserves a little before you start working on sleep. You are going to need the bandwidth to endure some freak-out. If you are twitching every time your child cries, let's take care of you first.

Feeling defeated

With the amount of determination livewires have, it's easy for parents to feel outmatched. We may set a boundary, but livewires are astonishingly capable of outlasting us. It's common for parents to feel like they don't have what it's going to take to stick by whatever limit they set. And then what happens? We relent, we cave, we wave a white flag—because whatever we were doing wasn't working anyway, and we're just so ridiculously tired that we can't withstand yet another meltdown today, so we'll just lie with them, give them a bottle, and read another book. *Anything* for a little more bed-time peace. I've seen many parents of livewires who have given up on even trying to set a limit because the fight is always too big and the likelihood of success always too small. Who can blame them? They're exhausted, shell-shocked from conflict, and not sure that fighting this latest battle will get them anywhere.

This is called *learned helplessness*, and it results from chronic unsuccessful attempts to change a negative situation. When you try and try to make a situation better and nothing works, you deflate and ultimately give up. A telltale sign for me is when parents say something like, *"I try to leave the room, but they won't let me."* These parents are saying that they *know* that the power dynamic is upside down, but they don't feel like they have the boatload of energy and commitment they will need to change it.

There's a level of defeat that I suspect many parents of livewires are living with—that no one talks about—and it takes a toll. The good news is that getting some traction on changing sleep behavior will show you that you *can* have an impact on your livewire's behavior and give you that little burst of "I've got this" that you may have been missing.

The ever-moving goal line and the ever-rising stakes

The boatloads of advice and knowledge that we have access to as modern parents have raised the bar even higher for parenting. Headlines convey the clear message that there is a minefield full of bad outcomes that parents can and should avoid—and that mistakes can have dire and lasting consequences. Parents start to think that if they make one false move, their child's future is toast, and they've made a mistake they can't ever fix. It's nuts. Rather than empowering parents with information, today's parenting advice often just ratchets up their anxiety, doubt, and worry.

The pressure is immense. And for parents of livewires, it's even worse. You are working hard to parent a child who's more challenging than the norm while reaching for a bar that is set impossibly high. This is a recipe for exhaustion and burnout. But I bet you know that already. We're going to talk about how to offload some of the pressure and expectations in chapter fourteen.

Very few ta-das

Parents of livewires don't get very many clear, in-the-moment wins. Especially in the first few years, you get very, very little feedback from your livewire that lets you know you're on the right track. *How do I know what's working at all? What if nothing is working? What if I've just been wasting my time?* (You're not wasting your time, I promise.) No matter how much good work you do with your sensitive, tantrum-y toddler, for example, they may still have just as many meltdowns. It may look like your efforts aren't landing. But that doesn't mean they aren't. It just means your livewire isn't showing it on the outside . . . yet.

It's easy to feel frustrated and discouraged because it looks like the crazy amount of effort you are putting into supporting and guiding and soothing (and not exploding yourself) is pointless. I promise, it's not. At all. Parenting a livewire requires a big chunk of pure faith that whatever we're doing *is* working and that the big payoffs will show up later. Trust me, they will.

Self-doubt

High stakes with few signposts that you're doing a good job does a number on parents' confidence. You may have tried a hundred different strategies to improve sleep (or other behaviors) that didn't work reliably and made you wonder if you have any kind of parenting instinct or ability at all. One of the most surprising findings from my parent survey was that, although parents of livewires were working so much harder, they thought they were doing a significantly worse parenting job.

"Every day, I worry that I'm not enough for her."

"I often wonder if what I experience is 'normal' and if I'm just not very good at parenting, since I seem to struggle so much more than other parents I know."

"This is my third child, and I have been VERY confident with raising my other two . . . but this one makes me feel like a first-time parent and more inept than I felt with my first child."

We're going to try to set this right if we can. It's incredibly easy to feel like the difficulties you are having with sleep and everything else are your fault or a reflection on your parenting skill. They aren't.

> **If you get nothing else from this book, I want you to know that no matter how you look at it, parenting a livewire is hard, and you are doing a great job, even when you don't feel like you are.**

Isolation

In many areas of the country, parenting young children can still be an isolating experience. If you don't live in a place with a lot of children or are somewhere that lacks gathering places (parks, parenting groups, etc.), you may really feel alone. Even if you have friends and family nearby, they may not understand or be able to handle your fussy baby or your sensitive toddler. Or they may like to offer all kinds of opinions that are not relevant or helpful for you. For parents of livewires, this sense that "I'm the only one with a child like this" is practically a given.

It's hard to feel like the odd one out—to have a child that just doesn't seem to track with what you are reading or seeing around you. You can feel very alone with it. But the fact that this book exists lets you know that you are not alone. There are lots of livewire parents struggling in isolation just like you are. The trick is to find the other parents who *are* on a similar path. They are out there. Find your people.

Stigma

Having a livewire can mean you feel like you're constantly under the parenting microscope because your child doesn't inhabit the world in the same way most other children do.

"We have six friends with children the same age or less than two months apart, and we are the ONLY ones whose child is not asleep before 8 PM. We are the only ones whose child must be held almost constantly. Everyone else's children sleep perfectly and play by themselves."

Having a livewire can also mean that you are apologizing or explaining a lot.

"They have trouble when they're overtired."
"They really just need a little time to warm up."
"They don't like it when strangers touch their hair."

And it's so easy to feel judged, especially during the dreaded public meltdowns. We worry what others think—we're "too permissive" or "don't know how to set limits." Or maybe others have even said as much.

"Feeling like we're failing or having a harder time as parents is not easy. Our friends and family who have easier babies tend to imply that we must be doing something wrong or that we should 'just try (whatever worked for them)' and cannot understand why that doesn't work with our son."

—Livewire parent of an eleven-month-old

The stigma of having a child that's not like most of the others their age can be painfully real. Any parent of a child who's different in some way experiences this. Ultimately, it just strengthens our resolve to fight that much harder for our unique child and to make the world understand their behavior rather than judge it.

Envy, resentment, loss

How many times have you heard someone say something like, "They're such a good baby. They started sleeping through the night at two months, and they've slept through ever since." Every parent of a livewire has a friend or two like this. The differences between the experiences of these parents and our experiences as parents of livewires couldn't be bigger.

I see this crop up whenever I do sleep talks for groups of new parents. Nine three- to four-month-olds will be lying happily on their blankets, playing or just hanging out while their moms chat and have snacks. And then there's that one tired parent in the back of the room bouncing her fussy little one—I'm sure wondering why her baby can't just lie there like the others so she can eat some goldfish crackers and talk like a grown-up for a minute.

In my survey, I asked parents to share three words that describe their experience of parenting their child. The words and phrases most used by parents of dandelions were "fun," "carefree," and "easier than I expected." *Not one* livewire parent used any of these words. They used words like "loving" and "powerful" but never "easy."

Coming face-to-face with the greener grass of parents with easier children is hard. While none of us would trade our livewires for anything, I'm sure we'd pay a small fortune to have the process be a little easier on us, at least some of the time. Feeling envious or grieving the loss of certain experiences is normal and comes with this territory. You wouldn't be human if you didn't have moments like this.

THE SURPRISING PERKS OF PARENTING A LIVEWIRE

Although we've spent a good chunk of time on the challenges, parenting a livewire does have deep and meaningful perks. If you are open to it, parenting a livewire puts you on a fast-track program of personal development. This is no yoga retreat in Mexico—this is an extreme growth boot camp. A livewire causes you to be a better parent—because you have to be. Livewires require (demand?) that you to step up and be *more* (patient, consistent, present, tolerant). They can stretch you to your limits, but just like any good workout, you build muscle in the process. If you are up for it, these kiddos make you a better human.

Self-awareness

Livewires force us to confront parts of ourselves that we could have easily and comfortably left stored in the shadows. In those raw, exhausted moments of parenting, the unfinished, unhealed parts of ourselves and any unresolved traumas we've locked away get triggered. If we pay attention to them—to those wounds that have been comfortably buried until now—we can see that these triggers might be signaling that parts of ourselves need acknowledgment and healing. Digging into the unhealed parts of our past is no fun and sometimes awful and messy, but it's also an incredible opportunity to stretch and grow.

I remember a particularly hard day when I shouted to the universe, "Why are my kids so *intense*?!" And then I had a crazy epiphany: "OMG . . . I think *I'm* intense." I honestly had no idea. I think I had just learned to *not* be intense (but I totally was). Learning about and loving my children's temperament gave *me* the opportunity to better understand myself and how I operate in the world . . . and that I'm not just weird. Without my livewires, I would have gone through life without really understanding that, apparently, I *too* am a livewire.

Radical acceptance

Life with a livewire means that your path diverges dramatically from the ones you read or hear about. It's different from potentially every parent friend you have. Yours is the child who gets overwhelmed at birthday parties. Yours is the child who won't just sit in the stroller while you have a chat. Yours is the child who has multiple meltdowns a day. Yours is also the child who's writing poetry at three or has full-on sentences by fifteen months. With most parents of children who don't quite fit the mold, there will be a moment when you are able to let go of the worry and accept that parenting is going to be different for you. You let go of what you *thought* it would be like and shift toward acceptance of how it *is* (and of all the wonderful chaos that entails).

> *"My therapist helped me reframe my parenting by internally saying, 'Thank goodness I am different.' I don't want to parent with harsh discipline or shaming. I choose to parent differently, and it IS often lonely—but thank goodness I am different. Thank goodness [my child] feels free to be a kid and express himself. While it is so hard every day, I am glad my son isn't put in this obedience / fear / compliance box like I was. I grew up afraid to mess up. He is free and loved and knows it."*
> —Livewire Mama, A. R.

Your child may never go to bed without talking to herself for forty-five minutes. Your child may never wear shirts with tags in them or have their food touching on their plate. You may not ever have a talk with your child where they look at you and say, "You're right. Thanks, Mom." (Maybe

when they're in their twenties and their frontal lobe has fully developed . . .
maybe.) But you *will* have your powerful, smart as a whip, empathic little
livewire who will fight you and surprise you and fill you up with joy.

Parenting a livewire means continually holding our livewires' better
angels in mind—even in the moments when it's really, really hard to do
that. We search for the reasons behind the screaming and meltdowns. We
try to avoid labeling them or blaming them. We believe in their goodness
despite the furious banshee they can be in the moment. It's an amazing
thing to be able to do for your little human . . . and if you can do this for
them, maybe you can do it for yourself a little, too.

Courage, commitment, and faith

It's one thing for you to be accepting of your livewire, but the world can be
another matter. Having a livewire means frequently having to advocate on
behalf of your very unique kiddo. Daycares, schools, and other social settings
are set up for dandelions because they make up the majority of children.
Makes sense . . . but it also means that parents of livewires often find themselves on the front lines, fighting for a better, more educated understanding
of their child. It's not always easy, and it also doesn't always feel great.

> *"This boy. The one who made me a mom. He is full of fierce fire. He's*
> *fun. He's fearless. But he is also obstinate, argumentative. He doesn't*
> *listen, and he pushes me to a level of despair I didn't know was possible.*
> *I'm constantly told he is too loud, too physical, too cheeky, too naughty.*
> *I support him, I advocate for him, I fight tooth and nail for my boy.*
>
> *But it's so lonely. When I share concerns with friends, I feel like*
> *it's my fault, I'm not strict enough, or I don't push hard enough. What*
> *I see as success is a failure for others.*
>
> *I constantly feel like I'm not enough and he's not enough."*
>
> —Livewire Mama, A. H.

It's so easy for these kiddos' behavior (or our parenting) to be misinterpreted. It's hard for anyone outside of the livewire tribe to understand. To many, our livewires are just "unruly" or "out of control." And we, as parents, are just "too permissive" or "helicoptering." Or there's the ever-popular "snowflake" label. As parents, we have to ignore it all and just forge ahead, knowing that our livewire is not like other children.

It's not easy. What's the line between responding to who our child is and just caving to it? I don't have the answer to that. Parents have to feel that out for themselves. I'm *still* trying to figure this one out. Parents of livewires often have to keep going despite whatever judgment or criticism or lack of understanding comes our way from others who think we're just not doing it right. This takes courage and faith and a willingness to look "wrong" to those who don't understand.

The opportunity to break the cycle

On top of a more difficult parenting road as a baseline, many livewire parents are also trying to give to their child what they themselves didn't get as children. Parents who were punished as a child for meltdowns strive to be present and understand the triggers of their livewire's emotional fireworks. Parents who were criticized because they were "too sensitive" strive to validate and support their livewire's sensitivity. Parents who were never allowed to "talk back" encourage their livewire's persistence and outspokenness. Parents who were spanked for misbehavior as children learn to discipline without it.

This is not easy. In fact, it is *much more work* to create new parenting pathways from nothing. You can't rely on your instincts because those may be rooted in your childhood. You have to learn new skills, read all the books, and retrain your brain to respond differently. Hacking out a new path that breaks family cycles of pain or dysfunction and gives your livewire what you needed but never got is nothing short of heroic.

THE RESULT OF ALL OF THIS? A CHRONICALLY EMPTY GAS TANK

I would say that the number one issue for parents of livewires is fatigue. Our work on sleep is going to help make a serious dent in your sleep debt. But even when your child is falling asleep at a reasonable hour, there are still chores to do or work to catch up on. Or maybe your child is finally sleeping, but *you* still can't. Managing the amount of investment livewires require, along with everything else it takes to make it through the day, can mean that you are chronically depleted. This fatigue takes its toll on your health, your relationships, and your parenting. If you are truly running on fumes, you should also know that you're not keeping that a secret. It probably shows.

Full disclosure: I had a lot of bad days when my children were little. *A lot.* I had two differently wired livewires who were twenty months apart, and I really, really wanted to do the best job I could for them. I wanted to validate how amazing they were and help them learn to navigate their powerful temperaments without them feeling "bad" or "wrong." I really wanted to do parenting *right*. But, good grief, was that a massive endeavor. It was so much harder than I ever imagined it could be, and many days, I just felt like roadkill.

I also knew full well that despite my best efforts to soldier through, my overwhelm and crushing fatigue still seeped out. How could it not? I was grumpy and so tired that I sometimes struggled to be present for them. How in the world was I supposed to help my children emotionally regulate when I felt like such a mess? Also, because I didn't know that I was a livewire, too, I had no idea how to navigate my own intensity. On bad days, my unaddressed intensity and sensitivity just busted out all over the place. Awful sleep issues with both of my children only made my lack of emotional regulation worse. Low on fuel, but still needing to keep moving up the steep and rocky road of each day, I just kept going—even when my engine was grinding so hard that smoke was billowing out from underneath the hood.

I would laugh when I saw advice like, *"Moms, take a time-out for a nice bubble bath."* Please. Like that was going to fix *anything*. There was not enough bubble bath in the world to make a dent in how exhausted I was. So, I rejected the idea as stupid and completely unhelpful. What I failed to realize was that, while a bubble bath wasn't a cure-all, it could have been a *cure-a-little*. More than twenty years down the road now, I can definitively say that rejecting *any* amount of self-care was a bad idea.

PARENTAL BURNOUT

Recent research has emerged about the serious consequences of parental burnout.[69] Parental burnout is defined as the reaction to a significant and chronic imbalance between resources (the gas in your tank) and demands (everything in your life that requires your full investment). It would not surprise me if *most* parents of livewires were at least burnout adjacent.

Researchers on parental burnout from the University of Louvain in Belgium looked at levels of cortisol (the stress hormone) in a large sample of parents and found that stress levels were *two times higher* in burned-out parents than in other parents . . . *and* higher than in adults with chronic severe pain.[70] Here's the kicker: Burnout can *cause* problems with sleep quality and quantity—not just the other way around.[71] Just like with your livewire, overtiredness can lead to less sleep, not more.

Burnout also has been shown to negatively impact parent-child relationships.[72] When stress is constant and parents don't have a way to refill their tanks, they may start pulling away from their child emotionally as a form of self-protection. Chronic demands on energy and time that continue past the point of needing a break can wear down our defenses. This is the point when we see our darker sides peek through, and we are not acting like the parent we really want to be.

HOW TO RECOGNIZE BURNOUT

Known indicators of burnout include:

- Brain fog
- Shorter temper
- Confusion
- Forgetfulness / difficulty remembering things
- Increased stress levels
- Depression
- Poor sleep (even when your child is sleeping)

If chronic stress and fatigue are not addressed and are allowed to continue, more serious symptoms include:

- Experiencing less pleasure in parenting
- Emotional distancing from children as a form of self-protection
- Feeling like you just aren't the parent you used to be or the parent you thought you could be
- In extreme cases, or in combination with other serious stressors, thoughts of escape (running away) or even self-harm / suicide

We have to take burnout seriously. It's not something you should just tough out—partly because of the mental and physical costs to you, but also because we can't hide it from our bright, perceptive livewires. It's important to acknowledge and accept the parts of this rodeo that you can't change, but you also have to commit to doing *whatever it takes* to bolster your energy and get some more gas in your tank. On this livewire journey, it's as important as making sure you eat and stay hydrated. In the next chapter, we are going to talk about steps you can take to reduce the load and refill your tank even a tiny bit. It may seem impossible at first to find any time for self-care, but there's a reason you always hear that darned preflight instruction to put on your own oxygen mask before helping others. The cost to your livewires of having a parent on the edge of collapse is real.

Remember, whatever place you are in right now, as you are reading this book, is okay. You are a rock star, and you are investing a ridiculous amount of commitment and effort in this work. Bravo, you. Now we need to get your reserves shored up so that you can keep going.

CHAPTER 14

Putting Some Gas in Your Tank: Snippets of Self-Care

There are so many ways that parenting a livewire zaps your personal resources. And that's *in addition* to running on so little sleep. Because it can be such a nonstop circus, finding a little recharge time can feel virtually impossible. You may have to get creative, and you may have to loosen your grip on some goals or standards to make it happen. Most importantly, you will have to commit to it. Because continuing to run on empty isn't an option. Your parenting and your mental health suffer when you are on the crumbling edge of burnout. Plus, there's no way you can be committed and consistent in your work on sleep coaching if your energy defenses are down. So, let's get you out of the chronic fatigue / burnout hole you are in because you are going to need your wits about you for tackling sleep (not to mention getting through childhood in one piece).

Getting you on a more even keel has two components: (1) *reducing your energy outflow* where you can, and (2) *filling up your reserves* with small moments of self-care.

REDUCING ENERGY OUTFLOW

When parenting small children, much of your energy outflow is non-negotiable. It has to happen. But there can be a host of ways that we add to that outflow by putting additional pressure on ourselves. Ask yourself whether there are ways that you are adding to your personal load that could potentially be released. Are there parts of your mindset that you can let go of to conserve your precious mental energy and start pulling yourself out of the burnout zone? How clean does the house have to be? Does that party really need a homemade cake? Will anyone actually suffer if you leave the house for forty-five minutes to take a walk by yourself?

Ditch the perfectionism and lower the bar.

The need to do it all "right" is a big contributor to burnout. Striving to always do the "best" possible thing (research based, responsive, authoritative, etc.) creates so much pressure. I know that if you are a smart, sensitive livewire parent, this "setting a high bar" is sort of your jam. You know how it *can* be or *should* be, so you strive to get there. You probably read everything you can get your hands on, and when it doesn't work with your livewire (because why would it?), you believe it's your fault. The fact that we can now track every moment of our livewires' days in terms of sleep and play and food and poop means that overachieving parents now have data to prove how they're not measuring up. Plus, in parenting advice, *success* is narrowly defined, and *screwing up* is not.

Here's the good news: This isn't how parenting works.

Even though it seems like you need to hit the bull's-eye in parenting every single time, you really don't.

Truly dysfunctional parenting is the result of repetitive patterns of problematic interactions—not merely veering off the path momentarily and having to course correct. That's normal parenting. It's how it's meant to be.

A lot of parenting advice makes it seem like you can prevent later problems if you do everything *just right* early on. Here's the hard truth: Even the best parenting will not inoculate your child against negative outcomes. There's a limit to what we can do to protect our kiddos. Life happens. Development happens. *Peers* happen. Your striving to do it all "right" won't prevent life from happening to your child.

So, *know* that you will make mistakes. *Big ones.* This is actually a good thing. Your children need you to be imperfect so they can learn that it's okay when *they're* imperfect. They need to see us screw up, take responsibility, course correct, and learn. Get good at making mistakes. Get good at being okay with it. You are doing your best with the information you have, and you are showing up and loving them and valuing them. Lower the stupid bar. (Or as the hilarious author Jen Sincero says, "Loosen your bone, Wilma.")[73] This is going to go for sleep, too. Where is "good enough"? It's okay for that to be your new bar.

You may also have to lower your expectations for a lot of your daily life. You may have to ditch the notion of your house being orderly or your child never watching a video or a million other "shoulds" because YOU HAVE A LIVEWIRE. Whatever you can do to make things easier or less stressful, you should absolutely do. You need every available brain cell and shred of energy just to keep your engine running. Think of this as *stamina conservation.*

Offload the load.

Partners can be amazing . . . *if we let them.* I've had many parents who come for sleep coaching where moms report doing every bedtime and all wake-ups. When I ask about the partner doing bedtime, they will tell me they tried it, but the baby cried a lot, so Mom came in and nursed. We have to give non-nursing partners the chance to figure things out, and let the baby figure the partner out.

In research, this effort to keep responsibilities under your own control and feeling overly anxious about others trying to help is called *gatekeeping.* It's common in moms, especially those who are really overtired. When you're exhausted, it often seems (and is) easier for you to just take care of the baby if you know there might be more struggle if you let your partner help. Moms are wired to respond strongly to their baby and to be really invested in the tasks of mothering. The all-consuming nature of the role can result in difficulty letting go of certain tasks and letting someone else help. Moms can worry that the other person won't do as good of a job or don't know as much as they do about what the child needs, or that the child might cry. Or maybe we just feel like it's our job to do it all.

Gatekeeping can not only directly contribute to high levels of fatigue and overwhelm but also prevent partners from developing the same kind of expertise and feeling of competence that moms get from all that practice. This can be especially true at bedtime. Partners can play a critical role in laying down new patterns with sleep—*but they have to have the opportunity to figure it out.* When one partner swoops in to rescue the other one, it ends up undercutting their confidence and conveying a lack of trust. The baby will be okay with a caring, involved partner. Breathe and let them have the opportunity to learn. Allowing help—even if it's not comfortable at first— has big, big payoffs for everyone involved.

Step away from the Instagram.

Social media can be a huge source of support. It can also be a source of anxiety, comparison, and feelings of not measuring up. Social media, in general, is a showcase for curated portrayals of parenting. It's easy to get the impression that other parents are having a much easier, more successful time than you are (plus, their hair looks better, and their houses are clean).

For most parents, the images we see on social media are unrealistic. For parents of livewires, it can be downright depressing. And I mean that literally. Studies have found that comparing oneself to images of parenting on social media is directly related to higher levels of depressive symptoms.[74] It's easy to get unrealistic impressions about what should be happening or what's expected. Comparing your own experience to the Insta-filtered micromoments of other people's lives and trying to keep up with those impossibly filtered images is not helpful and may make you feel worse than you already do.

If you need social media in your life, find a tribe of livewire parents with the same struggles you have. There, you will feel seen and supported, which will put gas *in* the tank rather than siphoning it out.

Release the need to have answers.

It's easy to feel like we're always supposed to know what to do as parents. With livewires, this just isn't remotely possible. We're not wizards. And neither is Google. In fact, searching the internet for answers often makes confusion and worry worse. Everyone has a solution and they're all different. Sometimes, the only solution is that there *isn't* a solution. Sometimes, the only option is to just be with your child as they are struggling.

This is important to keep in mind when it comes to bedtime distress, as they resist learning the go-to-sleep skill, but also for those meltdowns where there's nothing to be done but wait them out. We don't have to have a ready answer or perfect response. We can just be *with* them in our not knowing. We can offload that pressure to "do" something and, instead, just connect and be present. You don't have to fix anything. You can just be in the moment and release both you and your child from needing to be anything more.

REFILLING THE TANK: PUT ON THE DANG OXYGEN MASK

Cutting back on how we waste our emotional energy on worry and comparison is a good start to getting a little of our mojo back, but it won't completely solve the problem. In addition to conserving what you have, you will need to actively put energy back in your tank. When you are running on fumes, these actions should be priority one.

Take the dang bubble bath.

Even if you think that taking just a teeny break won't make a difference, do it anyway. This was my big mistake. I thought that because a small break wouldn't fix my exhaustion, why even try? Here's the thing: If you take a few moments to be alone even once a day, it *will* add up. And even more importantly, when you take a momentary break, you communicate to *yourself* that you deserve time and care. It may not do anything for you at first. You may need practice with taking a little care of you. Give it time.

You should shoot for at least forty-five minutes on your own each day, preferably out of the house but at least out of earshot of any children. It may sound impossible, but just do it. No one will suffer in forty-five minutes. Go on a walk. Go to the grocery store and just stare at all the kinds of shampoo for twenty minutes (this was my husband and me the first time Grandmama stayed with our first one). Get out of the house. Or, if you're an introvert, have your partner take your child or children out of the house, and you stay at home for some blessed alone time. Even if you don't believe it will do anything, there is literally no downside to trying.

Be your own Sherpa.

Remember when I talked about how crying and meltdowns can be triggering? For sensitive, empathic parents or those with past trauma or dysfunction, crying doesn't just set off an alarm—it triggers a full SWAT team of alarms. Personally, I get physically panicky when I hear a baby screaming in the grocery store. *Pick up the baby. Pick up the baby. PICK UP the BABY!!!* And then I have to leave the store. My system really reacts (and it isn't even my child!). I know this is true for a lot of parents. Crying can be physically and emotionally triggering. Parents will say, "We tried crying it out for like fifteen minutes, and I just couldn't do it . . . like, I *physically* couldn't do it."

Regardless of the reason, if your livewire's crying is physically or emotionally triggering, it's going to be difficult to think clearly, problem-solve, and then respond in a grounded way. Whether it's past trauma or anger and resentment bubbling up, when *we* are dysregulated by powerful feelings, our dysregulated child can't feel grounded or safe. It's sort of like when a little one falls. If the parent panics, the child also starts to panic. Little ones need *us* to be regulated so that they can eventually learn to regulate themselves. Emotional regulation starts with co-regulation. Our more mature nervous system provides an anchor and a map for our children when they have their big feelings. When we are in reactive mode and flooded with our own feelings, we aren't available to be that anchor. We cannot be their port in the storm if we are *also* lost in the storm.

Being able to remain calm and present while our livewires are losing it is an advanced-level skill. It's just not easy. If you're tired or overextended or dealing with past trauma, well, it's darned near impossible. It's like our defenses get worn down across the day until the nerve is totally exposed. I was always fine for the first few meltdowns in a day. I could be present and calm. But by the fifth or eighth one, I was a mess. I felt like I didn't know what I was doing. Nothing was working. I couldn't make it better or make it stop . . . and that made me angry at the universe for making this so hard . . . and then *I* was having a meltdown. Not fun.

So, what can you do to help yourself keep it together when your child is losing it (or you are)?

Dayna Abraham, author of *Calm the Chaos,* suggests an easy-to-remember three-step action you can take the minute you start feeling emotions start to boil over: stop, breathe, and anchor.[75]

Stop. Just having the presence of mind to say "stop" to yourself and acknowledge that you are starting to feel overwhelmed can be a huge part of short-circuiting your own freak-out.

Breathe. I know, I know. To me, this always sounded like a Band-Aid for a head wound. But deep, slow breathing is a science-based reset for your nervous system. When your alarm system has been triggered, you are firmly in your fight-flight-freeze mode, and there's no way you'll be thinking clearly. Take a deep, slow breath. Pause. Take another one.

Anchor. Be ready with a thought or affirmation that can zap you out of the unhelpful thoughts you might currently be having. Statements like

"My little one needs me" or "I don't have to be perfect in this moment" or "I don't have to know what to do right now" can help anchor you to the present and help switch you out of reactive mode.

When you're in a calmer place, you can also give some thought to whether there are particularly potent triggers that crop up a lot and what you might do to reframe them. Big feelings can happen in an explosive flash and we may not even be aware of what we're saying to ourselves that lights the match. If you start taking time to observe your own feelings and inquire about why they might be so big in those moments, you will learn more about the buried pain or need that's bubbling up.

Here's an example: You've been working and working to get your toddler's sixth meltdown of the day contained. It's dinnertime. You've tried everything you can think of, and the screaming and physical struggle is still going. You are tired and frayed. Suddenly, you feel furious—not just frustrated, *furious*. These are the moments when we know we are not our best selves. We may yell. We may have our own meltdown. Once you get through it (their meltdown and yours), can you do a little reflection about what's "up" for you in these moments? You may realize, for example, that every time you get really overwhelmed, you say to yourself, "OMG, why is this *always* so hard?!" or "Nothing I do works!" and that's what *really* lights the fury fuse.

If you take the opportunity to bravely look these triggers in the eye, you may realize that what you're feeling is a weight or wound that you have been carrying around for a while but haven't ever needed to confront. Now, because you're at such a low ebb energy-wise, you can't ignore it anymore. It has risen right up to the surface where you have to see it. The good news is that once it's in your conscious awareness, you can face it, reframe it, and ultimately release it. So, stop, breathe, and anchor in the moment, and know that these powerful feelings are actually opportunities for growth.

Lower the volume.

I have heard from many moms who swear by decibel-reducing earplugs. They do not block sound; they just reduce the volume of it. If you are auditorily sensitive and crying or yelling really triggers your nervous system, these may help a lot.

Build your village.

Support in whatever form you can access has been shown to dramatically reduce parental burnout and stress. Mental health support, partner support, friend support, mother-in-law support, support group support . . . all good. Get some.

Cut yourself some slack.

This is a biggie. Parents of livewires work so hard, often while thinking they're doing a terrible job. You are not doing a terrible job. This is just really, really tough. Do yourself a favor and try to practice self-compassion. which simply means turning toward yourself with kindness. This extremely simple action has been shown to be a powerful, powerful tool with all kinds of mental, physical, and emotional benefits.[76]

In any moment you are struggling or you feel like you're blowing it, take a deep breath, feel your feet on the floor (or otherwise ground yourself by holding your hands together, putting them on your chest, or feeling the chair underneath you), and acknowledge how hard you are trying and how committed you are to your livewire's well-being. Give yourself some credit for massively stepping up. Talk to yourself the way you would talk to a friend who was going through a rough patch. A mindfulness teacher I respect once told me that even if all you can do is say to yourself "There, there," it can still make a difference. You are doing your best in a very hard situation. Try to give yourself a little credit.

SEND UP A FLARE: WHEN IT'S MORE SERIOUS THAN "JUST TIRED"

Sometimes exhaustion can affect your emotions to a degree that it gets in the way of your ability to function, and you can't "just breathe" it away. It's important to let someone know that you are struggling before it gets bleak. With the availability of online therapy, virtual support groups, etc., there are more accessible options for mental health support today than ever before.

While mental health support can be helpful at any point, there are situations where it should be non-negotiable. Postpartum mood disorders are not limited to just depression or to just the first few months of parenting. Mental health challenges can happen any time—and *especially* when you feel exhausted. The links between sleep deprivation, parenting an intense child, and mood problems are documented and real.[77] The main indicator that tells you something needs addressing is that symptoms feel *out of scale* (bigger than the situation calls for) and *intrusive* (unwanted, persistent, and hard to ignore).

Postpartum Mood and Anxiety Disorders (PMADs)

What used to be considered primarily postpartum *depression* has now been expanded to encompass a range of mood disturbances. These are no longer limited to deep feelings of sadness or an inability to get out of bed, nor are they limited to biological parents. *All* parents can be vulnerable to emotional and mood changes after the arrival of a child. As with other "when to be concerned" questions, the key feature is that symptoms *get in the way of your daily functioning*, well-being, and ability to parent the way you'd like. If any of the following symptoms sound like you, get perinatal mental health support / evaluation and mention them to your doctor.

Postpartum depression

Postpartum depression (PPD) most often happens in the first few months after the arrival of a baby but can happen at any time in the first year (or beyond). Fathers and partners can also develop symptoms, but tend to develop them later than mothers—as late as twelve months postpartum—and their symptoms can differ. Also important to know: If one partner is depressed, the other partner is at a 50 percent risk of also developing a mood disturbance. All of this applies to same-sex and nonbiological parents (adoptive, surrogate) as well.

General PPD symptoms may include:

- Pervasive guilt and/or sadness.
- Losing interest in things you used to enjoy.
- Feelings of hopelessness.
- Big changes in eating or sleeping patterns (outside of caring for the baby).
- Inability to sleep (even when your child is sleeping) or sleeping too much.

Additional symptoms of PPD for men include anger, alcohol use, workaholism, impulsive / risky behavior, physical complaints (headache, digestive issues, etc.).

Postpartum anxiety

Postpartum anxiety (PPA) is considered by perinatal professionals to be even more prevalent than PPD and can include symptoms of obsessive-compulsive disorder or other anxiety-related conditions. However, because PPA can look a lot like normal, concerned, information-gathering parenting, it can be trickier to flag as something that needs attention. Two important indicators are that feelings are more intense than the situation warrants and that they feel intrusive or persistent. PPA symptoms may include:

- Racing thoughts.
- Near-constant worry.
- Feelings of dread about things you fear might happen.
- Worrying that terrible things will happen to the baby.
- Physiological symptoms (heart racing, shakiness, teeth grinding).
- Inability to sleep (even when your child is sleeping).

Postpartum rage

Yes, there's such a thing as *postpartum rage* (PPR). This is a relatively new category gaining attention from perinatal mental health professionals. PPR is not just an occasional response to frustration or fatigue or a moment when you temporarily lose it. Rather, it refers to a response that is disproportionate to the current situation and out of character. Symptoms include:

- Difficulty controlling your temper.
- Yelling and/or throwing things.
- Violent thoughts or urges.
- Feeling unable to snap out of it.

It may be difficult for you to tease out what is an actual mood or anxiety disorder and what is just the reality of trying to parent a livewire. In many ways, it doesn't matter. If you feel like things are unmanageable or you are not really yourself, send up a flare. It's a strength to ask for help, not a weakness. Reach out to a local perinatal mental health resource for assessment and support (make sure they have specific training in postpartum mood disorders).

TAKE TIME TO LOOK AT THE VIEW

This road can be steep. It can be long. Your muscles hurt, and you need a break and a snack. But if you don't consciously take a moment to appreciate how far you've come and the view from where you are, all you'll see, in the moment and looking back, is years of "hard." It's important to acknowledge what's working, what's surprising, what brings you a little joy.

How do you do that when you maybe aren't feeling it? Here's one super simple idea: Get a jar and cut some little scraps of paper. Each day (or whatever), write down something good and throw it in there. It can be tiny. I remember days when my gratitude thought was, *I like the way the milk swirls in my coffee in the morning.* When all else fails, you can be grateful for the things that *aren't* happening. You don't have a headache. The electricity is on. No one has the flu. We can always find *something* to be grateful for.

Gratitude helps us pay attention to the good that *is* in our day. Learning to notice and be grateful for even small, mundane aspects of life has been shown to have tangible effects on your mental health (including better self-esteem and well-being) and on your family.[78] And paying attention to what's good makes it easier to continue to find good in your day. Gratitude increases gratitude. Snippets of good (like snippets of self-care) can help you make it through the rough times.

Parents of livewires need to take their well-being seriously. Your livewire needs you to be on your game. If I could sit you down and put my hands on your shoulders, I would tell you this one thing that I wish someone had told me: Self-sacrifice is not the way to go. The parenting road is long and doesn't end with sleep training. Learn *now* how to carve out even a tiny bit of space for you and your well-being. You can't be the parent you want to be if you don't value yourself in the process.

CHAPTER 15

Reaching the Summit: The View from the Top

When your livewire is little, it can be difficult to think about *next week,* much less about when they're a young adult (and sleeping through the night). Given all the struggle, you may sometimes worry about how all of this will play out. It may sometimes feel like you're just trying and pivoting and trying some more, and you wonder if you're having any effect at all. It's like having planted seeds that just don't seem to be sprouting. You wait and work and worry. You water, you fertilize, you weed . . . and you think, *I'm pretty sure that if we did it right, we'd see <u>something</u> by now.* I promise, if it hasn't happened already, there *will* be a day when you start seeing little green shoots. Then, stand back and buckle up—because you didn't plant regular old seeds. These were some Jack and the Beanstalk–style *turbo-boosted* seeds: kaboom! A whole bumper crop of creativity, empathy, kindness, justice, ethics, courage, fearlessness, and astonishing understanding.

Even though your path feels longer and harder, I can tell you from a point farther down the road that it also comes with some *amazing* views— ones that you just will not see on an easier, more level trail. Trust me when I say that all the work and effort and tears you are putting into parenting now are going to pay off. If you can hold it together long enough to usher your livewire through their early intensity and sensitivity with grace and presence and just the right amount of firmness, they will grow into their livewire-ness without shame or the need to diminish who they are.

THE LONG VIEW: WHEN LIVEWIRES GROW UP

Parenting a livewire is a long game. So, even though this is a book about little livewires and sleep, and you are likely not thinking beyond the plateful of challenges you have right now, I wanted to give you a look at the long arc of this parenting circus—what happens *after* you get sleep handled and after the other twists and turns to come.

Parents of older livewires will tell you without hesitation that the effort you are putting into not squashing their spirit is totally worth it. Kim's and my livewires are all young adults now, and we can clearly see, despite all the chaos and tumult of those early years, the little breadcrumb trail of brilliance that led right up to the people they are today: creative, empathic, highly principled, ethical, intuitive, totally unique, and completely unafraid to speak their mind.

I sat down with a mom of two now-grown livewires, and she shared with me a little of her long view about one of them:

> I think that my daughter's temperament was really clear early on. And I was very thankful that I had some friends—strong feminist mother friends—that helped me to really trust that her energy, which was overwhelming (they all saw it, and they knew it was there, and they could see what a powerhouse she was), was a good thing. That it would eventually be a good thing. And so, there were many times where I had to kind of just trust that.
>
> And it's turned out to be true.
>
> Now, in her late twenties, she's working for a big advocacy organization. She's been promoted very quickly into upper management. And that grew out of a lot of the same stuff, the same impulses . . . wired for engagement, and a fearlessness . . . and rattling cages. Here was this

little kid who, to us, would stand her ground and say, "What are you going to do about it?" and now she's doing the same thing for a cause.

So, now, looking back, it really was the right impulse to trust that it would turn out okay. I would joke that the things that we are frustrated with at two years old are the things that we're going to really be blown away by at thirty. That ended up being very much the case with us.

I think that if there's any advice I'd give to people who are experiencing the same temperamental strength (particularly of their daughter), just to keep that unconditional love coming. It really does eventually pay off. And I will say that, even though we were not perfect parents, we didn't add on to it with more harm. You know what I mean? We kind of just took her as she was.

And sometimes we had some really difficult—really, really difficult—times. But now I know that even though it didn't seem like it ever would, it turned out okay. Better than okay. It definitely meant learning some new skills. But ultimately, you just love them whenever you don't know what else to do. Keep loving them through it. Just stick with it. There's going to be a place where this is all going to be okay.

Getting a livewire successfully to adulthood can be a long road with plenty of challenges. The challenges don't stop once they start sleeping . . . or go to school . . . or college. The challenges just change. Their heightened sensitivity can make them more vulnerable to a variety of emotional and psychological hurdles. They can be deeply affected by social dynamics and bullying in school. It can take less to really knock them on their butt, and they can have more trouble bouncing back. Remember when we talked about orchid temperaments that react much more strongly to such experiences? This is the reality of being a livewire.

Our work as parents is to help them steer their powerful emotions and brains while they develop resilience and coping skills. *Not easy.* We won't be able to protect them from negative events or experiences. We may not be able to prevent mental health challenges. All we can do is continue to understand both the upsides and challenges of the temperament hand they've been dealt and know that their difficulties can be a by-product of truly, truly profound depth and ability.

Remember that these sensitive children also react more strongly to supportive environments than mellower children. The work you are doing to support them and help them learn to manage their deep feelings will make a major difference in the long-term.

FAMOUS LIVEWIRES

It's easy to think that brilliant and creative people were always that way—old souls as babies, precocious as toddlers. But I am willing to bet, knowing what I know about livewires, that the vast majority of the most creative, gifted movers and shakers were a real handful as children. Albert Einstein was rebellious toward his teachers and other authority figures. Georgia O'Keeffe's sister said of her, "She had to have everything her way, and if she didn't, she'd raise the devil."[79] She was also known to be decisive in actions and beliefs, stubbornly insisting that God was female. Olympic gold medalist Michael Phelps, as a very young child, would ask "twenty-five zillion questions and always wanted to be the center of attention," according to his mother.[80] He had an extremely high energy level and though he struggled with maintaining focus and commitment in school, he was able to maintain intense discipline and drive in the pool. Amanda Gorman, poet and activist, was highly inquisitive and an overachiever at a very young age. She also experienced sensory processing difficulties and was self-admittedly stubborn. Her mother says she's always had intense levels of empathy and orientation toward social justice and she's never been afraid to stand up for what she believes.[81] Calm, cool Jackie Kennedy was also a livewire as a child. A teacher reportedly said she was "a darling child . . . very clever, very artistic, and full of the devil."[82] "Jackie was a rebel. She was brighter than most of her classmates and would get through her work quickly, then was left with nothing to do but doodle and daydream."[83]

Is it possible that the struggles you are having getting your livewire to sleep stem from a very powerful brain inside a tiny little body? Yes. Is it likely that this powerful brain will do big things when they're older? Also yes. Remember that parenting is a long game and that some of the challenging behaviors you're dealing with now will not be there for the long-term. Knowing that this chaos you're in right now will not last forever may help you cope a little. Your livewire may not win the Nobel Prize, but they will do something amazing—count on it.

A VOICE FROM THE FUTURE—OR, WHAT I WISH SOMEONE HAD SAID TO ME

Here are just a few nuggets of wisdom that I wish someone had told me back in the day.

> You can be confused.
> You can get it wrong.
> Parenting will suck.
> You may feel like you can't go on.
> > All of this is okay.
> You are doing hard, hard work.
> You are doing it because you value and respect your child's true nature.
> You are doing your best every single minute.
> You are taking leaps of faith constantly.
> > All of this is courageous and heroic.
> You can let things be "good enough."
> You can trust yourself to experiment and learn.
> You can give yourself a break because parenting is anything but straightforward.
> And when all else fails and you really, really don't know what to do . . .
> > Breathe . . .
> > and connect.
> > And just keep loving them through it.

ACKNOWLEDGMENTS

I'm so happy to have the opportunity to even write an Acknowledgments section. I'm so proud that this material went from "Someday, I should write a book about that" to . . . well, an actual book. I, of course, want to thank my coauthor, Kim West, who was the perfect bridge between my research, my parenting experience with livewires, and working with parents in a way that didn't involve cry it out. I keep thinking about how much different my own parenting journey would have been if I had met Kim then. I am so grateful to her for her openness and willingness to share in this book with me. I literally couldn't have done it without her (the book or my whole sleep / temperament career).

I'm also so grateful to Kim O'Hara, book coach extraordinaire, who held my feet to the fire to get the first manuscript draft completed in six months (a chapter a week!). This book would still be an incomplete list of bullet points on my computer's desktop if it hadn't been for my work with Kim O.

Thanks also to Leah Wilson, BenBella editorial rock star, who so kindly and so deftly helped shape this book. Her feedback and input were incisive, supportive, and sometimes hilarious. The whole BenBella team has been a dream to work with.

Thanks to the great professionals cited in the book and for their help reviewing pieces of the text for accuracy and relevance, including Cary Hamilton, LMHC, NCC, CMHS, RPT-S™, CDWF™ (child mental health

specialist); Dr. Whitney Cronin (naturopath); and Shoshana Bennet, PhD
(postpartum mood disorders expert). A special note of gratitude to Mary
Sheedy Kurcinka, PhD, whose book *Raising Your Spirited Child* I saw on
a bookstore display before I even had children and whose work on spirited
children was instrumental in parenting my own livewires (and realizing
that I'm one, too) and in how I approach and understand temperament.
She truly paved the path for a new way to think about challenging traits.

Lastly, I want to thank my own amazing, hilarious, brilliant parents—
who, I'm sure, are more livewire-like than they let on—and most importantly, my own family of livewires (every single one of us . . . even the
dogs): my incredible, force-of-nature daughter; my hilarious, deeply feeling
son; and my awesomely intense / sensitive husband, who's been with me on
every step of this crazy journey and has always encouraged me to be all of
myself. What a gift.

—Macall

A heartfelt big hug and thank-you to all the parents of livewires that I
have had the blessing of working with and learning from over the past
thirty years. Thank you for opening your hearts and allowing me to guide
and learn from you so that I could fine-tune the Shuffle and offer a gentle
approach for what I have called alert babies and children and now am calling livewires with Macall.

A thank-you to both my daughters for being unapologetically unique
and beautiful and teaching me to recognize and celebrate their individuality
and temperament from birth to forever. I love you to the moon and back.

It has been such an honor to work on this book with Macall. Her deep
understanding of research, temperament, and sleep, combined with her
funny, witty writing style (laughter can really help us get through the difficult moments of raising a livewire), and our shared experiences of raising
livewires, made this project so enjoyable and at times deeply moving. Working on this book with Macall has helped me to see the sensitive livewire in
me. The learning never ends! Thank you, Macall, for reaching out to me all
those years ago.

The BenBella team has once again been fantastic work with! It's been especially wonderful to work on this book with Leah, who has a livewire herself.

A big thank-you to Gretchen, my very own livewire, who taught me to be a better Sleep Lady and continues to teach me how to be a better mother and a loving, strong woman.

—Kim

NOTES

1. K. Spruyt, R. J. Aitken, K. So, et al., "Relationship Between Sleep / Wake Patterns, Temperament and Overall Development in Term Infants over the First Year of Life," *Early Human Development* 84, no. 5 (2008): 289–296, doi: 10.1016/j.earlhumdev.2007.07.002; B. M. Sorondo and B. C. Reeb-Sutherland, "Associations Between Infant Temperament, Maternal Stress, and Infants' Sleep Across the First Year of Life," *Infant Behavior & Development* 39 (2015): 131–135, doi: 10.1016/j.infbeh.2015.02.010.

2. N. Don, C. McMahon, and C. Rossiter, "Effectiveness of an Individualized Multidisciplinary Programme for Managing Unsettled Infants," *Journal of Paediatrics and Child Health* 38, no. 6 (2002): 563–567; M. D. Gordon, "The Effect of Difficult Temperament on Experiences with Infant Sleep and Sleep Training: A Survey of Parents," poster presented at the Occasional Temperament Conference, October 2020, University of Virginia.

3. W. T. Boyce, *The Orchid and the Dandelion: Why Sensitive People Struggle and How All Can Thrive* (New York: Pan MacMillan, 2019).

4. B. J. Ellis, T. Boyce, J. Belsky, M. J. Bakermans-Kranenburg, and M. H. Van Ijzendoorn, "Differential Susceptibility to the Environment: An Evolutionary–Neurodevelopmental Theory," *Development and Psychopathology* 23, no. 1 (2011): 7–28.

5. M. Pluess and J. Belsky, "Vantage Sensitivity: Individual Differences in Response to Positive Experiences," *Psychological Bulletin* 139, no. 4 (2013): 901.

6. Pluess and Belsky, "Vantage Sensitivity."

7. S. P. Batlivala, "Colic: An Evolutionary Selective Pressure for Good Parents?" *Clinical Pediatrics* 56, no. 8 (2017): 705–706, doi:10.1177 /0009922817696469.

8. A. Thomas and S. Chess, "The New York Longitudinal Study: From Infancy to Early Adult Life," in *The Study of Temperament: Changes, Continuities, and Challenges*, eds. R. Plomin and J. Dunn (Hillside, New Jersey: L. Erlbaum Associates, 1986): 39–52.

9. E. Aron, *The Highly Sensitive Child: Helping Our Children Thrive When the World Overwhelms Them* (New York: Harmony, 2002).

10. W. Sears and M. Sears, *The Fussy Baby Book: Parenting Your High-Need Child from Birth to Age Five* (New York: Little Brown, 1996).

11. M. S. Kurcinka, *Raising Your Spirited Baby: A Guide for Parents Whose Child Is More Intense, Sensitive, Perceptive, Persistent, and Energetic* (New York: William Morrow, 2022).

12. L. Budd, *Living with the Active-Alert Child* (Chicago: Parenting Press, 2003).

13. Lindsey Biel, email message to author, October 18, 2024.

14. Biel, email message.

15. M. Vasak, J. Williamson, J. Garden, and J. G. Zwicker, "Sensory Processing and Sleep in Typically Developing Infants and Toddlers," *The American Journal of Occupational Therapy* 69, no. 4 (2015): 6904220040p1-6904220040p8; K. Appleyard, E. Schaughency, B. Taylor, et al., "Sleep and Sensory Processing in Infants and Toddlers: A Cross-Sectional and Longitudinal Study," *American Journal of Occupational Therapy* 74, no. 6 (November / December 2020), doi: 10.5014/ajot.2020.038182.

16. V. Koshy and N. M. Robinson, "Too Long Neglected: Gifted Young Children," *European Early Childhood Education Research Journal* 14, no. 2 (2006): 113–126, doi:10.1080/13502930285209951.

17. A. Rastogi and M. D. Gordon, "Difficult or Gifted? Qualitative Investigation of Parents' Experiences of Their Gifted Children as Infants," poster presented at the Society for Research in Child Development Biennial Conference, March 22–24, 2019, Baltimore, Maryland.

18. S. Mendaglio and W. Tillier, "Dabrowski's Theory of Positive Disintegration and Giftedness: Overexcitability Research Findings," *Journal for the Education of the Gifted* 30, no. 1 (2006): 68–87.

19. L. H. Chadez and P. S. Nurius, "Stopping Bedtime Crying: Treating the Child and the Parents," *Journal of Clinical Child Psychology* 16, no. 3

(1987): 212–217; K. G. France, N. M. Blampied, and J. M. T. Henderson, "Infant Sleep Disturbance," *Current Paediatrics* 13, no. 3 (2003), 241–246, doi: 10.1016/S0957-5839(03)00004-6; V. I. Rickert and C. M. Johnson, "Reducing Nocturnal Awakening and Crying Episodes in Infants and Young Children: A Comparison Between Scheduled Awakenings and Systematic Ignoring," *Pediatrics* 81, no. 2 (1988): 203–213.

20. For solid, developmentally appropriate, non-parent-shame-y info on newborn sleep, check out *The Sleep Lady's Gentle Newborn Sleep Guide* (Dallas, Texas: BenBella Books, 2023).

21. L. J. Fangupo, J. J. Haszard, A. N. Reynolds, et al., "Do Sleep Interventions Change Sleep Duration in Children Aged 0–5 years?: A Systematic Review and Meta-analysis of Randomized Controlled Trials," *Sleep Medicine Reviews* 59 (2021), doi: 10.1016/j.smrv.2021.101498; J. Sleep, P. Gillham, I. St. James-Roberts, et al., "A Randomized Controlled Trial to Compare Alternative Strategies for Preventing Infant Crying and Sleep Problems in the First 12 Weeks: The COSI study," *Primary Health Care Research and Development* 3, no. 3 (2002): 176–183, doi: 10.1191/1463423602pc105oa.

22. I. St. James-Roberts, J. Sleep, S. Morris, et al., "Use of a Behavioural Programme in the First 3 Months to Prevent Infant Crying and Sleeping Problems," *Journal of Pediatrics & Child Health* 37, no. 3 (2001): 289–297, doi: 10.1046/j.1440-1754.2001.00699.x; R. Stremler, E. Hodnett, L. Kenton, et al., "Effect of Behavioural-Educational Intervention on Sleep for Primiparous Women and Their Infants in Early Postpartum: Multisite Randomised Controlled Trial," *BMJ (Clinical Research Ed.)* 346 (2013): f1164, doi: 10.1136/bmj.f1164.

23. D. G. Gee, "Sensitive Periods of Emotion Regulation: Influences of Parental Care on Frontoamygdala Circuitry and Plasticity," *New Directions for Child and Adolescent Development* 153 (2016): 87–110, https://doi.org/10.1002/cad.20166.

24. R. Feldman, C. W. Greenbaum, and N. Yirmiya, "Mother–Infant Affect Synchrony as an Antecedent of the Emergence of Self-control," *Developmental Psychology* 35, no. 1 (1999): 223.

25. C. B. Kopp, "Regulation of Distress and Negative Emotions: A Developmental View," *Developmental Psychology* 25, no. 3 (1989): 343–354, doi: 10.1037/0012-1649.25.3.343; L. A. Sroufe, "Early Relationships and the Development of Children," *Infant Mental Health Journal* 21, no. 1–2

(2000): 67–74, doi: 10.1002/(SICI)1097-0355(200001/04)21:1/2<67::AI
D-IMHJ8>3.0.CO;2-2.

26. I. Iglowstein O. G. Jenni, L. Molinari, et al., "Sleep Duration from Infancy
to Adolescence: Reference Values and Generational Trends," *Pediatrics* 11,
no. 303 (2003): 304.

27. A. S. Walters, D. Gabelia, and B. Frauscher, "Restless Legs Syndrome (Willis-
Ekbom Disease) and Growing Pains: Are They the Same Thing? A Side-by-
Side Comparison of the Diagnostic Criteria for Both and Recommendations
for Future Research," *Sleep Medicine* 14, no. 12 (2013): 1247–1252, doi:
10.1016/j.sleep.2013.07.013.

28. Dr. Whitney Cronin, email message to author, March 12, 2024.

29. A. Kahn, M. J. Mozin, E. Rebuffat, et al., "Milk Intolerance in Children with
Persistent Sleeplessness: A Prospective Double-Blind Crossover Evaluation,"
Pediatrics 84, no. 4 (1989), 595–603; O. Bruni, S. Sette, M. Angriman, et
al., "Clinically Oriented Subtyping of Chronic Insomnia of Childhood," *The
Journal of Pediatrics* 196 (2018): 194–200.e1, https://doi.org/10.1016/j.jpeds
.2018.01.036.

30. Dr. Whitney Cronin, email message.

31. T. Banzon, D. Y. Leung, and L. C. Schneider, "Food Allergy and Atopic
Dermatitis," *Journal of Food Allergy* 2, no. 1 (2020): 35–38.

32. M. Romanos, A. Buske-Kirschbaum, R. Fölster-Holst, et al., "Itches and
Scratches: Is There a Link Between Eczema, ADHD, Sleep Disruption
and Food Hypersensitivity?" *Allergy* 66, no. 11 (2011): 1407–1409, doi:
10.1111/j.1398-9995.2011.02705.x.

33. M. Castejón-Castejón, M. A. Murcia-González, J. L. Martínez Gil, et al.,
"Effectiveness of Craniosacral Therapy in the Treatment of Infantile Colic:
A Randomized Controlled Trial," *Complementary Therapies in Medicine*
47 (2019): 102164, doi: 10.1016/j.ctim.2019.07.023; H. Haller, G. Dobos,
and H. Cramer, "The Use and Benefits of Craniosacral Therapy in Primary
Health Care: A Prospective Cohort Study," *Complementary Therapies in Medicine* 58 (2021): 102702, doi: 10.1016/j.ctim.2021.102702.

34. M. Müller, A-L. Zietlow, E. Tronick, et al., "What dyadic reparation is meant
to do: An association with infant cortisol reactivity," *Psychopathology* 48,
no. 6 (2015): 386–399.

35. P. Fonagy and M. Target, "Attachment and Reflective Function: Their Role in Self-organization," *Development and Psychopathology* 9, no. 4 (1997): 679–700.

36. N. Jian and D. M. Teti, "Emotional Availability at Bedtime, Infant Temperament, and Infant Sleep Development from One to Six Months," *Sleep Medicine* 23 (2016): 49–58, https://doi.org/10.1016/j.sleep.2016.07.001.

37. R. L. Gómez, R. R. Bootzin, and L. Nadel, "Naps Promote Abstraction in Language-Learning Infants," *Psychological Science* 17, no. 8 (2006), 670–674, doi:10.1111/j.1467-9280.2006.01764.x; A. Hupbach, R. L. Gomez, R. R. Bootzin, et al., "Nap-Dependent Learning in Infants," *Developmental Science* 12, no. 6 (2009): 1007–1012, doi: 10.1111/j.1467-7687.2009 .00837.x.

38. M. Balbo, R. Leproult, and E. Van Cauter, "Impact of Sleep and Its Disturbances on Hypothalamo-pituitary-adrenal Axis Activity," *International Journal of Endocrinology* 2010 (2010).

39. Marie-Hélène Pennestri, email message to author, December 2, 2022.

40. B. C. Galland and E. A. Mitchell, "Helping Children Sleep," *Archives of Disease in Childhood* 95, no. 10 (2010): 850–853.

41. G. E. Quinn, C. H. Shin, M. G. Maguire, et al., "Myopia and Ambient Lighting at Night," *Nature* 399, no. 6732 (1999): 113–114.

42. K. Zadnik, "Association Between Night Lights and Myopia: True Blue or a Red Herring?" *Archives of Ophthalmology* 119, no. 1 (2001): 146.

43. K. R. Simon, E. C. Merz, X. He, et al., "Environmental Noise, Brain Structure, and Language Development in Children," *Brain and Language* 229 (2022): 105112, doi: 10.1016/j.bandl.2022.105112.

44. S. A. Hong, D. Kuziez, N. Das, et al., "Hazardous Sound Outputs of White Noise Devices Intended for Infants," *International Journal of Pediatric Otorhinolaryngology* 146 (2021): 110757, doi: 10.1016/j.ijporl.2021.110757.

45. A. D. Staples, C. Hoyniak, M. E. McQuillan, et al., "Screen Use Before Bedtime: Consequences for Nighttime Sleep in Young Children," *Infant Behavior & Development* 62 (2021): 101522, doi: 10.1016/j.infbeh.2020.101522.

46. E. M. Cespedes, M. W. Gillman, K. Kleinman, et al., "Television Viewing, Bedroom Television, and Sleep Duration from Infancy to Mid-Childhood," *Pediatrics* 133, no. 5 (2014): e1163–e1171.

47. S. I. Greenspan and N. Lewis, *Building Healthy Minds: The Six Experiences That Create Intelligence and Emotional Growth in Babies and Young Children* (New York: Da Capo Lifelong Books, 2009); F. Roghani, M. Jadidi, and J. Peymani, "The Effectiveness of Floortime Play Therapy on Improving Executive Functions and Cognitive Emotion Regulation in Children with Attention Deficit / Hyperactivity Disorder (ADHD)," *International Journal of Education and Applied Sciences* 2, no. 4 (2022): 30–44.

48. A. De Grauwe, J. K. M. Aps, and L. C. Martens, "Early Childhood Caries (ECC): What's in a Name?" *European Journal of Paediatric Dentistry* 5 (2004): 62–70.

49. B. A. Moore, P. C. Friman, A. E. Fruzzetti, et al., "Brief Report: Evaluating the Bedtime Pass Program for Child Resistance to Bedtime—A Randomized, Controlled Trial," *Journal of Pediatric Psychology* 32, no. 3 (2007): 283–287, doi: 10.1093/jpepsy/jsl025.

50. S. W. Garber, R. F. Spizman, and M. D. Garber, *Monsters Under the Bed and Other Childhood Fears: Helping Your Child Overcome Anxieties, Fears, and Phobias* (New York: Villard, 2011).

51. J. Cantor, *Mommy, I'm Scared: How TV and Movies Frighten Children and What We Can Do to Protect Them* (San Diego: Harcourt, 1998).

52. L. Sayfan and K. H. Lagattuta, "Scaring the Monster Away: What Children Know about Managing Fears of Real and Imaginary Creatures," *Child Development* 80, no. 6 (2009): 1756–1774, doi: 10.1111/j.1467-8624.2009.01366.x.

53. J. D. Woolley and H. M. Wellman, "Origin and Truth: Young Children's Understanding of Imaginary Mental Representations," *Child Development* 64, no. 1 (1993): 1–17, doi: 10.1111/j.1467-8624.1993.tb02892.x.

54. Sayfan and Lagattuta, "Scaring the Monster Away."

55. Sayfan and Lagattuta, "Scaring the Monster Away."

56. Sayfan and Lagattuta, "Scaring the Monster Away."

57. Sayfan and Lagattuta, "Scaring the Monster Away."

58. W. L. Mikulas, "Graduated Exposure Games to Reduce Children's Fear of the Dark," in *Behavioral Treatments for Sleep Disorders*, eds. M. Perlis, M. Aloia, and B. Kuhn (Elsevier, 2011): 319–323, doi: 10.1016/B978-0-12-381522-4.00033-X.

59. J. Sommers-Flanagan and R. Sommers-Flanagan, *How to Listen So Parents Will Talk and Talk So Parents Will Listen* (Hoboken, New Jersey: John Wiley & Sons, 2011).

60. S. Blunden, J. Osborne, and Y. King, "Do Responsive Sleep Interventions Impact Mental Health in Mother / Infant Dyads Compared to Extinction Interventions?: A Pilot Study," *Archives of Women's Mental Health* 25, no. 3 (2022): 621–631.

61. Jian and Teti, "Emotional Availability at Bedtime," 49–58.

62. Blunden, Osborne, and King, "Do Responsive Sleep Interventions," 621–631; M. R. Gunnar and C. E. Hostinar, "The Social Buffering of the Hypothalamic-Pituitary-Adrenocortical Axis in Humans: Developmental and Experiential Determinants," *Social Neuroscience* 10, no. 5 (2015): 479–488, doi: 10.1080/17470919.2015.1070747.

63. A. W. Van Meijeren-van Lunteren, T. Voortman, M. E. Elfrink, et al., "Breast-feeding and Childhood Dental Caries: Results from a Socially Diverse Birth Cohort Study," *Caries Research* 55, no. 2 (2021): 153–161.

64. K. F. Davis, K. P. Parker, and G. L. Montgomery, "Sleep in Infants and Young Children: Part Two: Common Sleep Problems," *Journal of Pediatric Health Care* 18, no. 3 (2004), 130–137, doi: 10.1016/S0891.

65. Davis, Parker, and Montgomery, "Sleep in Infants," 130–137.

66. S. Bhargava, "Diagnosis and Management of Common Sleep Problems in Children," *Pediatrics in Review* 32, no. 3 (2011): 91–99; Davis, Parker, and Montgomery, "Sleep in Infants," 130–137; A. K. Leung, and W. L. Robson, "Nightmares," *Journal of the National Medical Association* 85, no. 3 (1993): 233; A. K. Leung, A. A. Wong, A. H. Hon, et al., "Sleep Terrors: An Updated Review," *Current Pediatric Reviews* 16, no. 3 (2020): 176–182.

67. A. P. Wagner, *Worried No More: Help and Hope for Anxious Children*, 2nd ed. (Apex, NC: Lighthouse Press, 2005).

68. S. Maushart, *The Mask of Motherhood: How Becoming a Mother Changes Our Lives and Why We Never Talk About It* (New York, Penguin: 1999).

69. M. Mikolajczak, J. J. Gross, and I. Roskam, "Parental Burnout: What Is It, and Why Does It Matter?" *Clinical Psychological Science* 7, no. 6 (2019): 1319–1329.

70. M. E. Brianda, I. Roskam, and M. Mikolajczak, "Hair Cortisol Concentration as a Biomarker of Parental Burnout," *Psychoneuroendocrinology* 117 (2020): 104681.

71. A. Sarrionandia-Pena, "Effect Size of Parental Burnout on Somatic Symptoms and Sleep Disorders," *Psychotherapy and Psychosomatics* 88 (2019): 111–112.

72. A. Gillis and I. Roskam, "Daily Exhaustion and Support in Parenting: Impact on the Quality of the Parent–Child Relationship," *Journal of Child and Family Studies* 28, no. 7 (2019): 2007–2016, doi: 10.1007/s10826-019-01428-2.

73. J. Sincero, *You Are a Badass: How to Stop Doubting Your Greatness and Start Living an Awesome Life* (New York: Running Press, 2013).

74. J. E. Sidani, A. Shensa, C. G. Escobar-Viera, et al., "Associations Between Comparison on Social Media and Depressive Symptoms: A Study of Young Parents," *Journal of Child and Family Studies* 29, no. 12 (2020), 3357–3368.

75. D. Abraham, *Calm the Chaos: A Failproof Road Map for Parenting Even the Most Challenging Kids* (New York: Simon Element, 2023).

76. F. M. Sirois, S. Bögels, and L. M. Emerson, "Self-Compassion Improves Parental Well-Being in Response to Challenging Parenting Events," *Journal of Psychology* 153, no. 3 (2019): 327–341, doi: 10.1080/00223980.2018.1523123; K. D. Neff and D. J. Faso, "Self-Compassion and Well-Being in Parents of Children with Autism," *Mindfulness* 6, no. 4 (2015): 938–947, doi: 10.1007/s12671-014-0359-2.

77. M. E. McQuillan and J. E. Bates, "Parental Stress and Child Temperament," in *Parental Stress and Early Child Development: Adaptive and Maladaptive Outcomes*, eds. K. Deater-Deckard and R. Panneton (New York: Springer, 2017): 75–106.

78. S. K. Nelson-Coffey and J. K. Coffey, "Gratitude Improves Parents' Well-Being and Family Functioning," *Emotion* 24, no. 2 (2024): 357–369, doi: 10.1037/emo0001283.

79. R. Robinson, *Georgia O'Keeffe: A Life* (Waltham, Mass.: Brandeis University Press, 2016).

80. M. Winerip, "Phelps's Mother Recalls Helping Her Son Find Gold-Medal Focus," *New York Times*, August 8, 2008, https://www.nytimes.com/2008/08/10/sports/olympics/10Rparent.html.

81. T. Drinks, "Amanda Gorman, Youth Poet Laureate, Has Speech and Auditory Processing Issues," https://www.understood.org/en/articles/amanda-gorman-youth-poet-laureate-has-speech-and-auditory-processing-issues.

82. A. S. Malkus, *The Story of Jaqueline Kennedy* (New York: Grosset & Dunlap, 1967).

83. A. Hunt and D. Batcher, *Kennedy Wives: Triumph and Tragedy in America's Most Public Family* (New York: Lyons Press, 2014).

ABOUT THE AUTHORS

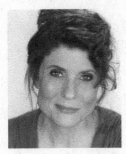 **Macall Gordon** is a researcher, speaker, and certified Gentle Sleep Coach with twenty years of experience examining parenting advice on infant sleep and how it impacts parents and children. She has a master's degree in applied psychology from Antioch University Seattle with a research-based specialization in infant mental health and sleep. She also has a BS in human biology from Stanford University, where she specialized in the interplay of biology and culture. She has conducted and presented research on sleep training advice, parental experiences with sleep training, the "bright sides" of temperament, and how that impacts sleep at infant and child development conferences around the world. She has also led advanced training for sleep coaches, mental health providers, and others on temperament and sleep. She is the director of the Fussy Baby Site, a support resource for parents (facebook.com/thefussybabysite). She comes to this work because she had two sensitive, alert, intense children (now young adults), and she didn't sleep for eighteen years. Find out more about Macall on her website (littlelivewires.com) or on social media (@littlelivewires).

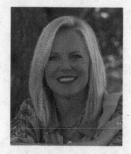

Kim West, MSW, is a mom of two who has been a practicing child and family social worker for over twenty-five years. She has personally helped over twenty thousand families all over the world gently teach their children how to fall asleep—and fall back asleep without leaving them to cry it out alone. She started training Gentle Sleep Coaches internationally in 2010 and has appeared as a child sleep expert in numerous magazines and newspapers, and on television programs including *Dr. Phil*, *TODAY*, and *Good Morning America*.

More Sleep Support

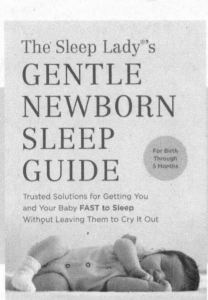
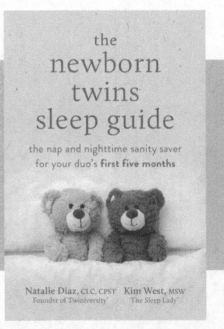
Available now where books are sold.